Behavioural changes associated with pain
in companion animals

For this English edition:

Behavioural changes associated with pain in companion animals

Plaza Antonio Beltrán Martínez nº 1, planta 8 - letra I
(Centro empresarial El Trovador)
50002 Zaragoza - Spain

D.L.: Z 1821-2012

Design, layout and printing:
Servet editorial - Grupo Asís Biomedia, S.L.
www.grupoasis.com
info@grupoasis.com

Warning:

Veterinary science is constantly evolving, as are pharmacology and the other sciences. Inevitably, it is therefore the responsibility of the veterinary surgeon to determine and verify the dosage, the method of administration, the duration of treatment and any possible contraindications to the treatments given to each individual patient, based on his or her professional experience. Neither the publisher nor the author can be held liable for any damage or harm caused to people, animals or properties resulting from the correct or incorrect application of the information contained in this book.

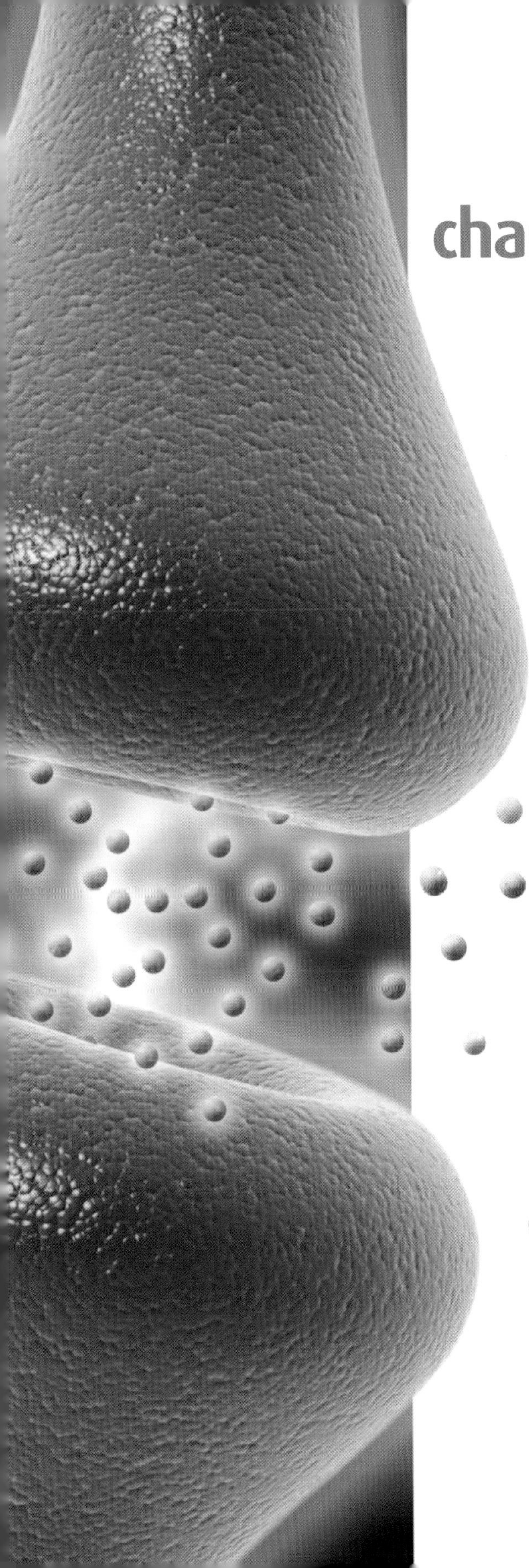

Behavioural changes associated with pain

in companion animals

Tomàs Camps Morey

Marta Amat Grau

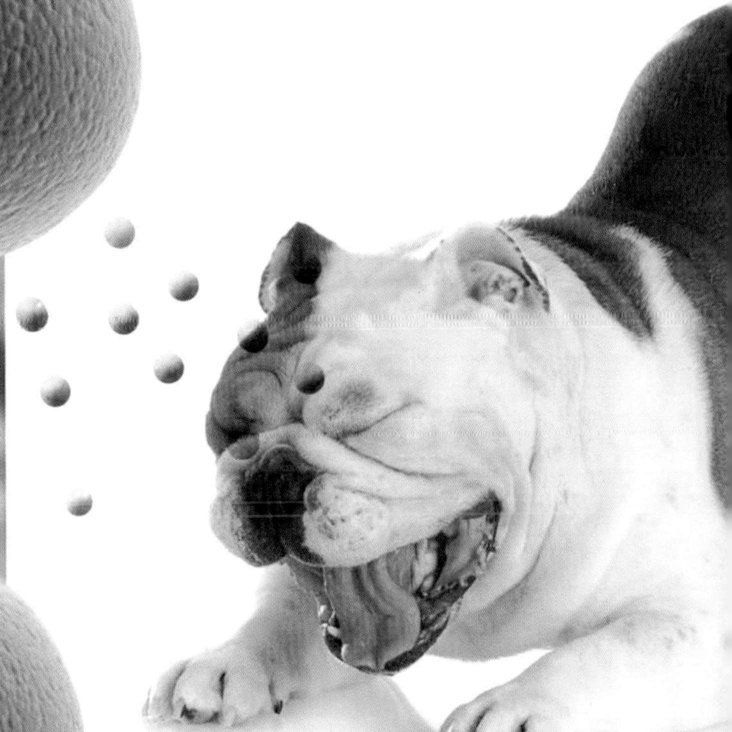

SERVET

I would like to thank Xavier for his patience and valuable advice, Marc Vallori (r. i. p.) for teaching me animal respect and giving me my first book about animal behaviour at the age of 14. I would also like to thank my parents for always believing in me and for the effort they made so I could follow my career path, my brother and sister for their support, Spud for keeping me company over the past 12 years and finally, I would like to thank Joana, for always being there, understanding me and bearing me.

Tomàs Camps

I would like to thank my parents and my children, Pol y Alba, their support has made the hard task of reconciling work and family easier. I would like to thank Xavi for encouraging me during all this time and always being at my side. And I would like to take advantage of this opportunity to thank my dogs Shadow and Flor and my cat Maruru for their company. Thank you with all my heart.

Marta Amat

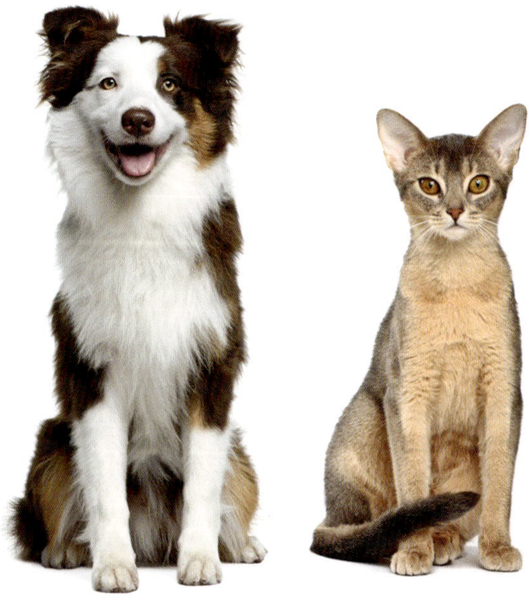

Authors

Tomàs Camps Morey

Graduated in Veterinary Medicine from the Autonomous University of Barcelona (UAB) in 2004. Master's degree in Clinical Ethology by the UAB in the same year. He has been a Diplomate of the ECAWBM -European College of Animal Welfare and Behavioural Medicine- since 2011. He was in charge of a private clinical animal behaviour service for four years.

Since 2009 he has been part of the Nutrition and Animal Welfare Service (SNIBA, *Servicio de Nutrición y Bienestar Animal*) of the UAB. He is also a veterinary surgeon at the Ethology Service of the UAB Veterinary Clinical Hospital and has been president of the Clinical Ethology Group of the Spanish Association of Veterinary Surgeons Specialised in Small Animals (GrETCA, *Grupo de Etología Clínica de AVEPA*) since 2002.

Marta Amat Grau

PhD in Veterinary Medicine. Diplomate of the ECAWBM, European College of Animal Welfare and Behavioural Medicine.

Veterinary surgeon at the Ethology Service of the UAB Faculty of Veterinary Medicine Clinical Hospital since 2001. Head of the Ethology Service since January 2009.

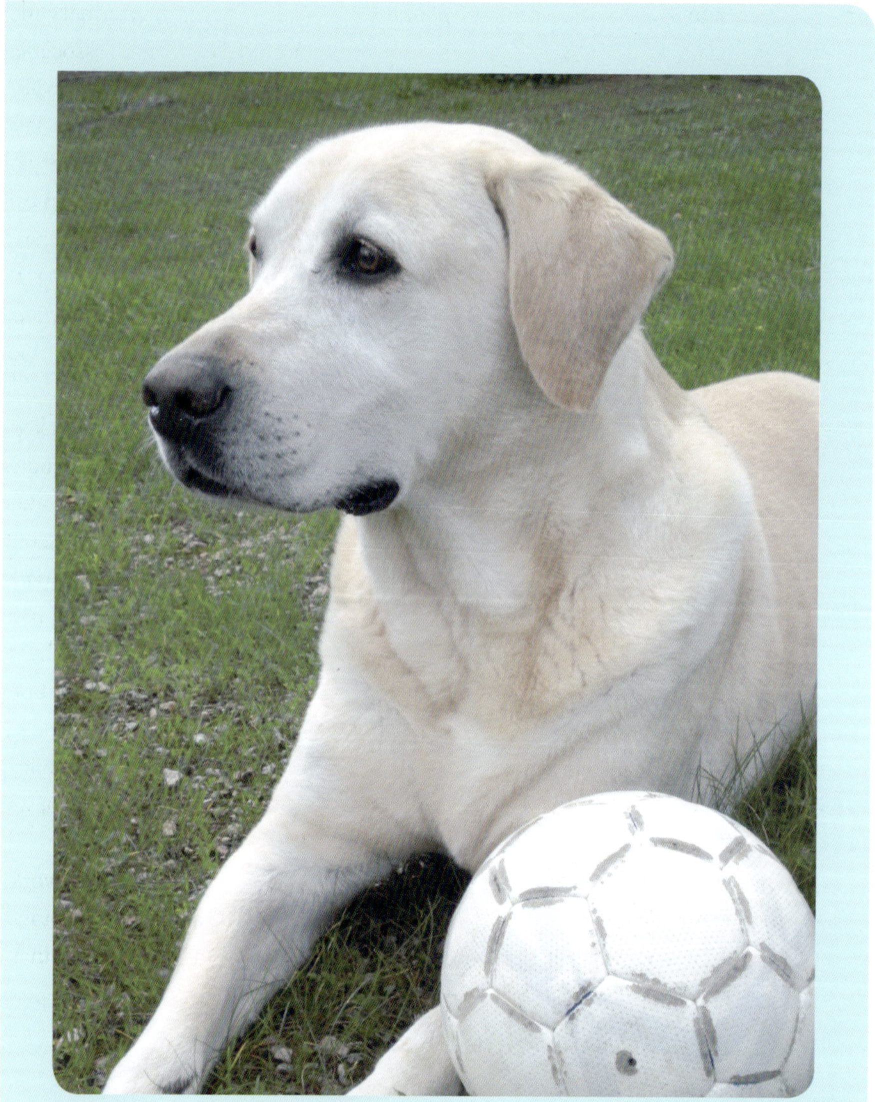

Foreword

The treatment and prevention of pain are essential elements in veterinary medicine. Pain -which is defined as an unpleasant emotional experience associated with tissue damage- is an important cause of suffering in animals and professional ethics thus obliges us to do our best to reduce our patients' pain. Furthermore, pain triggers a stress response which can complicate the recovery of an animal that is sick or has undergone a surgical procedure. Finally, pain can contribute to the manifestation of problematic behaviours - such as aggressive behaviour - which not only reduce the satisfaction derived from owning an animal but also have negative consequences on both the animal and its owners' welfare.

Fortunately, the use of analgesics to reduce pain in animals that are sick or have undergone surgery is more and more frequent. However, various studies conducted in different countries indicate that analgesics are still not as widely used as desired. Although this is probably due to a combination of reasons, one of them is the lack of rigorous, easily accessible information with an essentially practical approach that could help the vet to identify the manifestations of pain and choose the best strategy to prevent or reduce it. In addition, it is still relatively common to find members of the veterinary profession with ideas about pain in animals which are in clear contradiction with the scientific evidence that has been gathered in the past few years. For all these reasons, the publication of a quality book about pain in companion animals is always good news.

This book has several characteristics that differentiate it from other works about pain in companion animals. One of them is that the authors have known how to explain both the fundamental and most practical aspects of pain in an

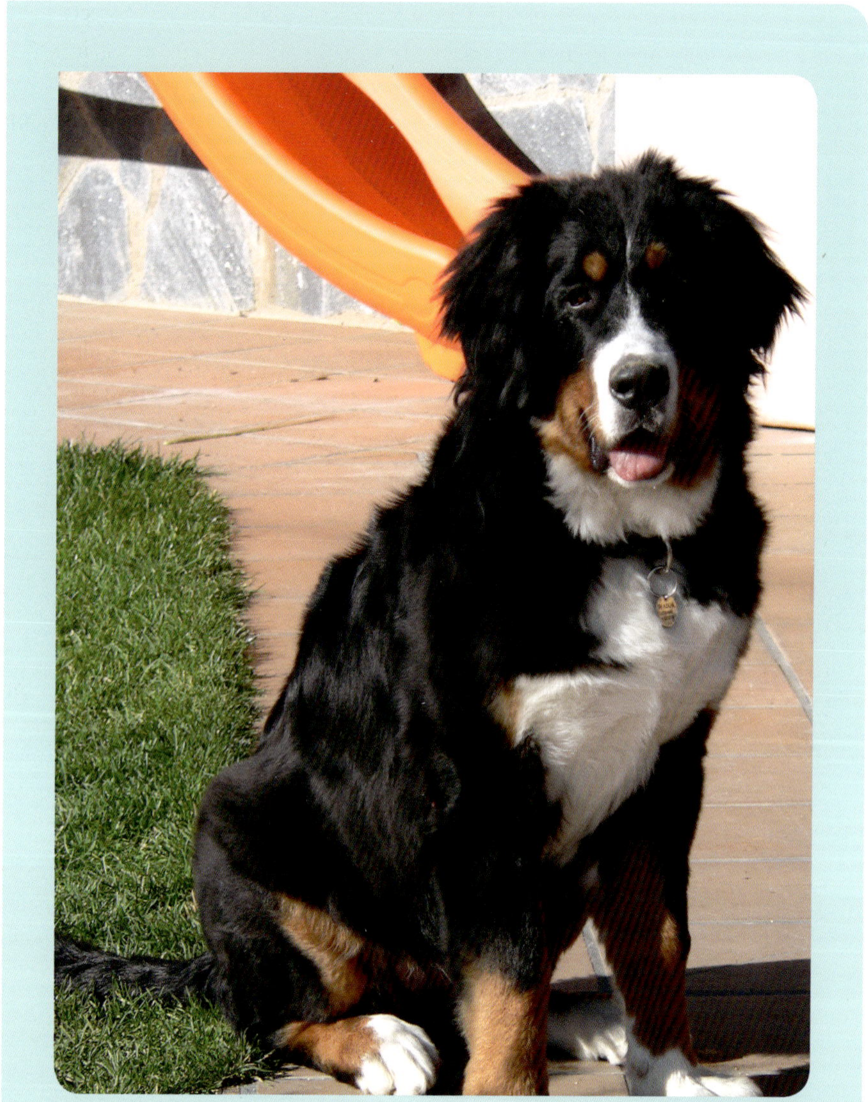

easily understandable language. Including essential aspects of the physiology of pain and the mechanism of action of analgesics is, in my opinion, truly important. Indeed, an approriate clinical training cannot be based on memorising diagnostic or treatment protocols. It must include the understanding of the basic mechanisms which explain these procotols. This allows practictioners not only to understand the reasons for carrying out certain diagnostic or therapeutic procedures, but also to modify their protocols according to each patient's needs.

Furthermore, the authors have included aspects which, although they are very important, are not usually mentioned in most books about pain. These aspects include, for example, a discussion of the concept of animal welfare and its importance in small animal medicine, as well as a review of the behavioural changes caused by pain in dogs and cats.

In conclusion, the book that is now in the reader's hands will no doubt contribute to improving the training of clinical vets in all the aspects related to pain in small animals. I am convinced that reading it will benefit both veterinary surgeons and their patients. The broad clinical experience of the authors and their sound academic background are the best guarantee of that.

Xavier Manteca Vilanova
PhD in Veterinary Medicine
Professor of Animal Behaviour
Master's degree in Applied Animal Behaviour and Animal Welfare
Autonomous University of Barcelona

Table of contents

GENERAL CONCEPTS AND PHYSIOLOGY OF PAIN

General concepts

Definition of pain and nociception

According to the International Association for the Study of Pain (IASP), pain is "an unpleasant sensory and emotional experience associated with actual or potential tissue damage". It is a mechanism of protection that involves physiological and behavioural changes, whose role is to reduce or avoid tissue damage and promote the animal's recovery.

In general terms, it includes four basic elements:

- **Transduction:** it is the conversion of the noxious stimulus (which can be thermal, physical or chemical) into a nerve impluse. It takes place in the nociceptors, which are the receptors in charge of receiving the painful stimulus.
- **Transmission:** it is the propagation of the nerve impulse, generated in the nociceptors, to the central nervous system (CNS).
- **Modulation:** it refers to the adjustment of the nerve signal intensity, and thus the pain intensity, mediated mainly by the endogenous analgesia system.
- **Perception:** this is the final process which takes place in the brain and causes the subjective and unpleasant feeling that is specifically termed pain. It is the emotional or affective aspect of pain.

Nociception differs from pain as it refers only to the "physiological or sensory process involved in the painful experience". It is the identification or detection of a harmful or potentially harmful stimulus. It therefore lacks the emotional or affective component.

In other words, pain refers to the general process of the painful experience and includes both physical and emotional feelings and responses. On the other hand, nociception could be measured by quantifying the electrical and chemical activity of the neurons involved and, if there was no emotional component, would be fairly proportional to pain.

Both the physiological and behavioural changes associated to pain can be measured to assess pain in animals. However, it must be taken into account that while physiological changes are very similar among the different species, behavioural changes can vary greatly among species and among individuals of the same species.

The fact that there are species in which those behavioural changes are subtle, in addition to the fact that animals do not have the verbal capactity to express themselves, led for many years to the thought that animals did not have the ability to feel pain.

History of pain in animals. Are they able to experience pain?

Nowadays, most of the scientific community accepts the fact that animals, at least mammals and birds, are able to experience pain. However, it has not always been the case. Historically, the attitude towards animals has been that of considering them as machines or simple automatons that do not have reason and are unable to feel pain and suffering. This idea was defended by great scientists and philosophers in history, such as Descartes (1596-1650), who said that "the greatest prejudice of our childhood is to believe that animals think", as well as "emotions - we must remember that by definition pain has an emotional component - are exclusive to human beings".

Although such an opinion can nowadays seem obsolete, the methodological, and even conceptual, difficulties raised by the study of pain in animals should not be forgotten.

In order to understand these problems better, it is important to remember the four phenomena that take place when experiencing pain. Three of those four components, transduction, transmission and modulation, are relatively easy to study objectively by means of methodologies typical of physiology. However, the same does not happen with the fourth phenomenon, perception, since it involves an affective or emotional component that, by definition, is a subjective experience that cannot be observed directly. On the other hand, it is the affective component that is critical from an ethical point of view. If we came to the conclusion that there is no such emotional component, we would have no ethical responsibility to prevent or treat it, since pain as a cause of suffering in animals would not exist.

Jeremy Bentham (1748-1832) was one of the first philosophers who questioned the ideas defended by Descartes. He claimed that 'the question is not, "Can they reason?" nor, "Can they talk?" but rather, "Can they suffer?". There are various reasons why it is now accepted that animals can experience pain and suffering and, therefore, an affirmative answer can be given to the question raised centuries ago by Bentham.

The main reason is the so-called **principle of analogy**. According to this principle, animals are able to experience pain and suffering since the structures of the central nervous system (CNS) in charge of feeling pain and other forms of suffering in humans, are very similar to those of animals. Although people and most animals differ in some very specific aspects of the CNS, the areas and functions of the CNS that are necessary to experience suffering are very similar in many vertebrates. In addition, animals respond in a very similar way to humans in situations in which we feel pain and suffering. It is therefore more than reasonable to think that animals have the ability to feel pain and other types of suffering if we consider that the responses of their nerve structures are similar.

Another reason why it is difficult to think that the ability to experience pain is exclusive to humans is the so-called **evolution argument**. Taking into account that the ability to feel pain is an evolutionary advantage that helps the individual who has it to avoid real or potential risks, it is difficult to think that it appeared spontaneously in human beings without being present, in a more or less developed form, in other animals.

There is other evidence in favour of animals being able to feel pain:

- The first is that they are able **to learn how to avoid painful stimuli.** It is very common in the consulting room to see dogs trying to avoid at all costs a situation which turned out to painful for them on a previous occasion (for instance administering an injectable product). Many studies show that animals are able to learn how to avoid a painful stimulus and learn to show both withdrawal reflexes and complex avoidance behaviours, for example, with rats capable of jumping over obstacles to avoid electric shocks.
- Another proof is that they **learn how to self-administer analgesia.** This fact has been shown both in laboratory rodents and chickens, in studies in which it was observed that they learnt to self-administer analgesics when they suffered from tissue damage while they did not do so if there was no such damage. Furthermore, the amount of analgesics self-administered depends on the intensity of the pain felt.
- Finally, the last argument is based on the fact that the behavioural changes associated with pain are less marked when the animal is in a **new environment.** According to some authors, this would suggest that distractions brought by the new environment make the animal become temporarily less aware of pain. This effect would not be observed if pain was a mere reflex response without the emotional component.

Lastly, some authors defend that, even if all those arguments were not convincing enough, we should give animals the **benefit of the doubt**, and treat them as if they really had the ability to suffer.

Is it important to prevent and treat pain in animals?

The prevention and treatment of pain in pets are important for several reasons:

- It is a welfare issue (this aspect is defined in chapter 4).
- It can alter basic physiological functions that will have an effect on the individual's health: reduced food intake, immunological competence, etc.

Veterinary medicine and pain: treatment and prevention

In spite of accepting the fact that animal can feel pain in a similar way to human beings and that, moreover, pain affects the well-being of animals, the truth is that the use of analgesics in animals is much lower than it should be.

Surgical procedures without any analgesia are frequent in production animals. As an example, a study showed that approximately 80% of male piglets are castrated without any analgesia annually in the USA.

We must not fall into the error of thinking this problem is only found in the field of animal production. A study carried out at the end of the 90s with 2,000 English small animal veterinary surgeons (Capner C.A. et al., 1999), analysed their attitude when administering perisurgical analgesia in dogs, cats and small mammals. The study revealed that 97% of the vets gave analgesia for orthopaedic procedures in dogs. However, only 53% administered analgesia for ovariohysterectomies and 32% for orchiectomies. In the case of cats, the percentages were even worse. 94% administered analgesia for orthopaedic surgeries, but only 26% did so when neutering females and 16% with males. In the case of small mammals (hamsters, guinea pigs, rabbits...), although 93% of the vets claimed they carried out surgical procedures, only 22% administered analgesics routinely (fig. 1). An interesting data from the study was that women and young vets were much more prone to administering analgesics than men and older graduates. Another similar study conducted in Canada among 275 veterinary surgeons (Dahoo S.E. and Dahoo I.R., 1996), over the same period of time as the study previouly mentioned, showed very similar results in the percentages of administration of analgesics.

Figure 1. Results of a study conducted in the United Kingdom about the percentage of vets who administer analgesics in dogs, cats and small mammals (Capner C.A. et al., 1999).

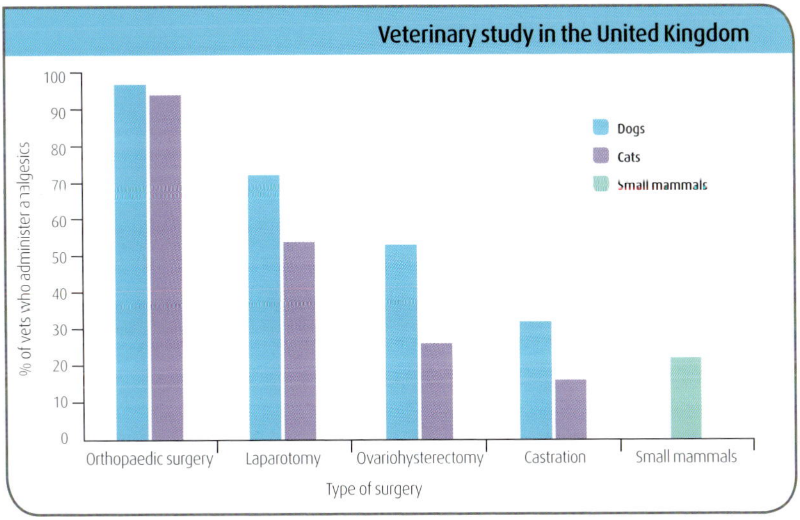

Myths about analgesics

Although these figures are likely to be much higher today than the ones given here thanks to the greater awareness and more extensive training of vets in this field in the past ten years, there are still some myths about analgesics that translate into a relatively high percentage of cases in which pain is not treated properly:

- **Some species feel less pain than others:** there is a belief that some species feel less pain than others. As mentioned previously, the neural pathways in charge of detecting noxious stimuli are very similar among species, at least among mammals and birds. This leads to thinking that it is very likely that animals experience similar levels of pain when faced with the same stimulus. It is often said that herbivores (companion animals such as rabbits and guinea pigs, but also production animals such as domestic ruminants for example) are less sensitive to pain than carnivores. This statement is false and does not have any scientific basis. What really seems to occur is that some species are more stoic than others when it comes to expressing their pain. Some authors have suggested that the species that are usually the prey of predators tend to express less pain since they would be an easy target for predators if they did so. The fact that they express less pain, however, does not mean in any way that they feel it less.
- **Pain can be beneficial to recovery:** a British study showed that 30% of vets believe that "animals need to feel a certain intensity of pain so that they are not too active after surgery". This myth probably comes from the concept that pain is biologically beneficial and has a protective function. Indeed, when an animal feels pain, it prevents it from using the affected area in order to avoid more tissue damage. However, it is important to point out that in clinical conditions, in which it is possible to control most of the variables, eliminating pain, and therefore its protective biological effect, is not a disadvantage, but rather the opposite. It has been shown that the advantages of eliminating pain exceed the alleged beneficial effect it has. Various studies show that an inadequate pain control delays both the healing and general recovery of the animal, in addition to increasing the risk of sepsis.
- **Analgesics hide the physiological signs of deterioration in hospitalised animals:** there is a false belief that some analgesics, such as opiates, hide some symptoms normally used by clinicians to detect a deteriotation of the health of critical patients, such as increased respiratory and heart rates in

hypotonic and hypoxic animals. The evidence, both in humans and animals, seems to indicate that it is not the case. Although it is true that opiates can potentially cause bradychardia, it has been proved that, even when they are administered in high doses, the heart continues to respond well to hypoxia, hypovolaemia and hypercapnia. If we also consider that with the use of opiates, the vet will eliminate pain as a cause of tachycardia, not only will the signs of deterioration not be hidden, but they will be even more obvious.

Why do vets administer less analgesics than they should?

Apart from the three myths that have just been mentioned, there are other reasons why vets keep administering less analgesics than they should:

- **Difficulties to identify pain in companion animals:** identifying and, even more, quantifying pain in animals is not easy. A wrong identification will translate into a lesser use of analgesics to prevent it and treat it. How to identify pain in companion animals will be analysed in the next chapters.
- **Control of narcotics:** some analgesics used in veterinary medicine, such as morphine, require a strict legal control through the use of narcotic prescriptions and a safe storage, due to their potential use as abuse drugs in humans and their addictive effect. This extra control represents an obstacle for some vets to use it on a routine basis.
- **Choice of the appropriate analgesic:** the range of analgesics available for use in animals is very wide and constantly increasing. As there are more options, continuous professional training in this field will be necessary in order for vets to feel confident when using analgesics and to avoid any reluctance due to the lack of information about active substances. The different groups of analgesics, their characteristics and possible interactions with other drugs used for behavioural problems will be analysed later on.
- **Side effects:** every drug has potential side effects and analgesics are not an exception. The risks of their use should always be evaluated against their benefits. These risks can be reduced by choosing the right analgesic for each particular case, and in these cases, the benefits are usually greater than the risks.

- **Cost of analgesics:** many professionals tend to reduce the cost of their procedures so that their clients are satisfied with the service provided, perhaps influenced by the competition from their colleagues. The use of analgesics obviously has a cost, and therefore, some veterinary surgeons could be prejudiced when having to administer them, in order not to increase the costs for the owner and thus avoid losing a client. On many occasions, however, this choice is made without asking the owners whether they are willing to pay for those costs. Whatever the reason may be, this translates into a poorer analgesia for animals.

Continuous training for professionals of the sector (veterinary surgeons, nurses, etc.) would help to eliminate those myths, thus helping to improve the use of analgesics in companion animals.

1

Physiology of pain

As already mentioned several times, pain has a physiological component (nociception), that includes the processes of transduction, transmission and modulation, and an affective or emotional component, which is called perception (fig. 2).

Figure 2. Diagram of the structures involved in the descending modulation of the painful signal.

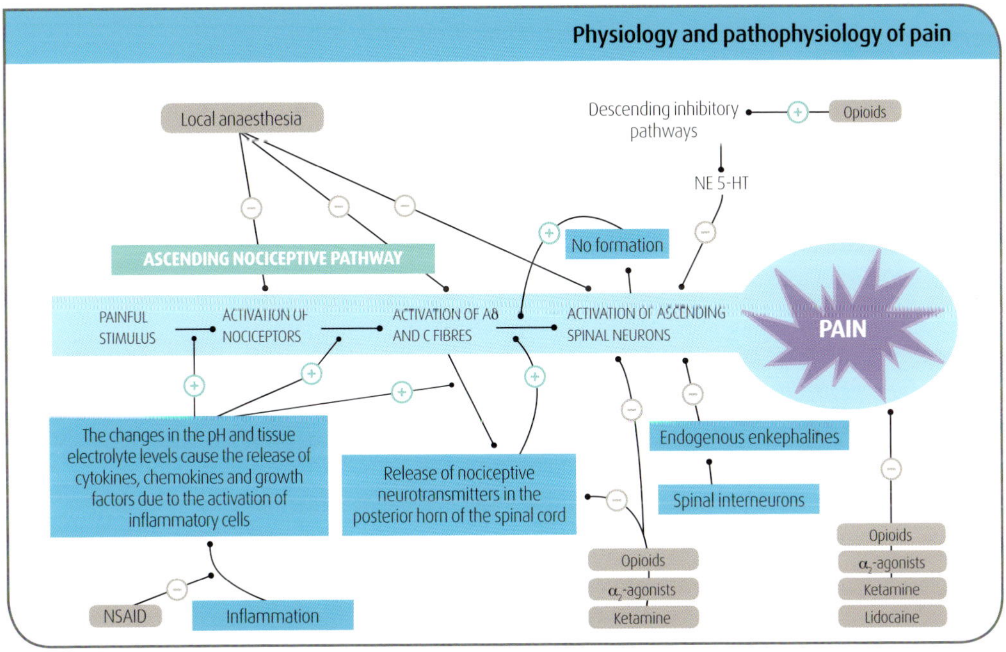

Extracted from: Driessen, B., Zarucco, L. Pain: From diagnosis to efective treatment. *Clinical Techniques in Equine Practice*, 2007; 6(2):126-134.

Transduction

The first process of nociception is transduction. Its purpose is to turn noxious stimuli into an electric signal. These stimuli can be thermal, mechanical or chemical.

Pain receptors are the axonal endings of neurons located in the posterior horn of the spinal cord. These neurons are called **first-order neurons**. Nociceptors are found in the skin, peritoneum, pleura, periosteum, subchondral bone, articular capsules, blood vessels, tendons, fasciae and internal organs. Noxious stimuli cause the opening of the nocicepive ion channels producing the nerve impulse, which can be continuous or intermittent. The more intense the stimulus will be, the more intense the impulse and the more frequent the bursts of impulses will be.

There are two types of nociceptors, **Aδ fibres**(A delta fibres) and **C fibres:**

- **Aδ fibres:** they respond to noxious, or potentially noxious, mechanical and thermal stimuli. They are myelinated fibres of large diameter that transmit the information at a high speed (5-30 m/s). As a result, Aδ receptors are responsible for what is known as first pain. They produce an acute, well-located and temporary signal. They will have a direct reaction with reflex responses.
- **C fibres:** they mainly respond to mechanical and chemical stimuli. They can also respond to thermal stimuli if they are extreme. They are non-myelinated fibres of small diameter that conduct the stimuli at a slow speed (0.5-2 m/s). They intensify the signal generated by the Aδ receptors and the sensation resulting from their stimulation is more diffuse and prolonged. The feeling of pain remains even once the noxious stimulus has stopped. They are responsible for the so-called **second pain** or **slow pain.**

To summarise, these two types of fibres, with their different speeds of conduction and stimulation properties, can explain the biphasic pain response that the reader will have probably experienced after a painful stimulus: a first sharp and localised pain that is followed by a diffuse pain with a burning sensation. In addition, the density of receptors in each location can also explain the different types of pain we experience. As an example, the density ratio of Aδ/C receptors in the skin is 1/2, while in internal organs this ratio goes from 1/8 to 1/10, which explains why visceral pain is much more difficult to locate than when there is a skin lesion.

Both Aδ and C receptors have a common characteristic: their stimulation threshold, under normal conditions, is high -although there are some differences according to their location (for example, mechanical corneal receptors have a lower stimulation threshold than the skin)-. This means that low-intensity thermal, mechanical or chemical stimuli are not going to activate them and they are therefore not going to generate pain. Only when the stimulus is very intense, and thus likely to cause tissue damage, are the receptors stimulated and pain is felt.

Finally, there is one last type of receptors involved in the general pain response, those composed of **Aβ fibres**, also called **mechanoreceptors**. They are myelinated fibres that transmit the impulse at a high speed (30-70 m/s) and their stimulation threshold is very low. They will therefore be activated by stimuli that, because of their low intensity, do not activate Aδ and C receptors. As a consequence, these fibres will be in charge of receiving the information from stimuli such as touch, pressure, vibration and joint movement. Although these receptors are not directly related to the generation of the painful impulse, they are linked to its modulation (which will be analysed later on).

Transmission

First-order neurons will form synapses with **second-order neurons**, which are also located in the grey matter of the spinal dorsal horn. There are various types:

- **Inhibitory or excitatory interneurons:** they will be involved in the process of pain modulation in the spinal cord.
- **Neurons responsible for reflex responses:** as a consequence of pain, such as withe withdrawal of the extremities for example.
- **Neurons responsible for the reflex sympathetic response:** they are responsible for the vascular changes associated with tissue damage, such as vasoconstriction, and for the release of noradrenaline in the damaged tissue area.

- **Projection neurons:** they transmit the information from the nociceptors towards the brain. There are three different types:
  - **Nociceptive-specific second-order neurons: they only receive information from** Aδ/C fibres. They are mainly located in somatic areas. Their basic function is to locate pain topographically in the body.
  - **Second-order wide dynamic range (WDR) neurons:** they receive information both from Aδ/C fibres and Aβ receptors. The information they receive converges from large areas of the body and is generated both in the somatic and visceral areas.
  - **Complex neurons:** they receive both somatic and visceral information.

All these neurons are involved in the initial processes of modulation, processing and integration of pain. They will help to provide an organised response to pain.

Projection neurons send the information to the brain and are organised in three tracts or pathways:

- **Spinothalamic tract:** involved especially in the conscious localisation of pain, the characterisation of the noxious stimulus and the emotional or affective response. It is the most important pain pathway in the spinal cord. It ascends towards the thalamus.
- **Spinoreticular tract:** part of the neurons from this pathway reach the thalamus and the activating reticular system (ARS). The spinoreticular tract is involved in the emotional response to pain, such as anxiety and suffering, and is repsonsible for the inhibitory effect that pain has on sleep and even, on the depth of anastesthesia. The ARS controls the level of activation of the CNS and is therefore related to the sleep- wake cycles, as well as the response to anaesthetics. Pain activates the ARS, which would explain how pain interferes with sleep. It would also explain why the anaesthetic depth can be reduced as a consequence of pain with a poor intraoperative anaesthesia.

The spinoreticular pathway is also an important descending pathway of the endogenous modulation system (which will be analysed further on).

- **Spino-hypothalamic tract:** it is mainly involved in the hormonal response associated with pain (such as the stress response for example).

Perception

It is difficult to define exactly at which level of the CNS the nociceptive signal is perceived as pain and causes suffering. This emotional or affective component, which we previously called perception, is the result of the activity of various brain structures:

- **Medulla oblongata, pons and mesencephalon:** they contribute to perception by connecting the ARS with the periaqueductal grey (PAG).
- **Reticular formation:** it receives information from various brain areas. It seems to have a crucial role in the integration of the painful experience since noxious stimuli have a very marked effect on reticular neuronal activity. It projects fibres to the thalamus and limbic system. It has an important effect on both the affective and motivational components of pain. This latter refers to the commencement of voluntary movements as a response to the pain signal.
- **Periaqueductal grey (PAG):** it is very important in the descending modulation of pain.
- **Hypothalamus:** it integrates both neuronal and hormonal information.
- **Thalamus:** it mediates in some aspects of the sensory discrimination of pain (nature of the pain) as well as in affective and emotional aspects.
- **Limbic system:** it mainly mediates in the emotional and motivational components of pain.
- **Brain cortex:** it has an important role in the anticipation of pain, the learning processes related to painful experiences and the associations that are established. It is capable of adjusting the negative emotional response (unpleasant sensation) and mediates in complex behavioural responses.

Modulation

Animals have an intrinsic analgesic system that inhibits ascending pain messages and their perception by means of descending signals. Various structures are involved in this process: the brain cortex, thalamus, PAG, pons and spinal dorsal horn neurons.

The PAG receives descending information from the cortex, the amygdala and the thalamus. The result of this stimulation is the release of endogenous opioids with an analgesic activity. In addition, as previously mentioned, both excitatory and inhibitory neurons that modify the intensity of pain perception can be found in the spinal cord. In short, the magnitude of the pain signal that will finally reach the brain and give rise to the actual pain would be the sum of:

- The signal from nociceptors.
- The signal from the endogenous control system.

The modulation process of pain signals in the spinal cord by means of descending messages from the brain and local inhibition, through the action of interneurons, is known as the **gate control theory**. This theory was proposed more than 45 years ago (Melzack and Wall, 1965).

According to them, the signal that reaches the brain is the sum of various effects, both inhibitory and excitatory. In order to understand the process, it is necessary to mention the elements that play an important role in it: **second-order neurons**, which are located in the grey matter of the spinal dorsal horn, receive information from Aδ/C **nociceptors** and Aβ **mechanoreceptors**, as well as information from **inhibitory and excitatory neurons** which, in turn, receive **descending (inhibitory) information** and are also connected with Aδ/C and Aβ fibres (remember that Aβ fibres are activated by inocuous stimuli such as touch and vibration, and that Aδ/C fibres have a high stimulation threshold).

If a second-order neuron receives a signal from Aδ and C fibre nociceptors, it will start to discharge, and the signal will be increased by the excitatory interneuron, but will then be adjusted by the descending inhibitory signal. The resulting final signal that will reach the brain will therefore be the sum of all these influences (fig. 3).

Figure 3. Diagram I of the gate control theory (Melzack and Wall, 1965).

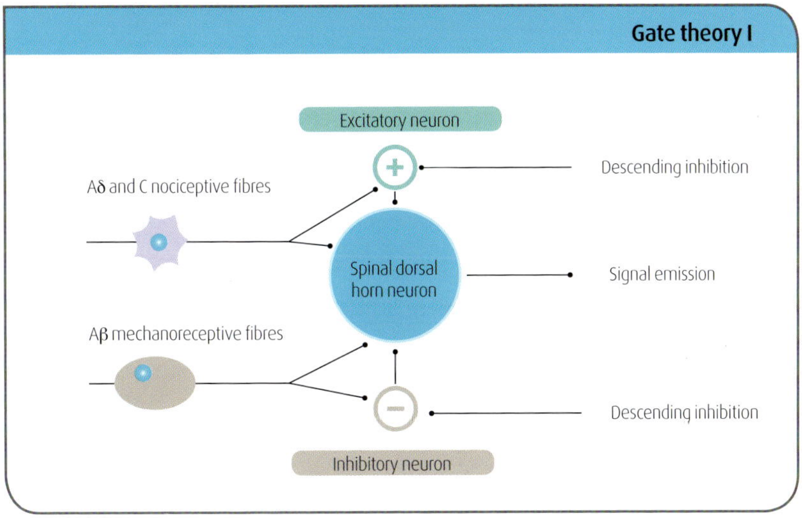

Figure 4. Diagram II of the gate control theory (Melzack and Wall, 1965).

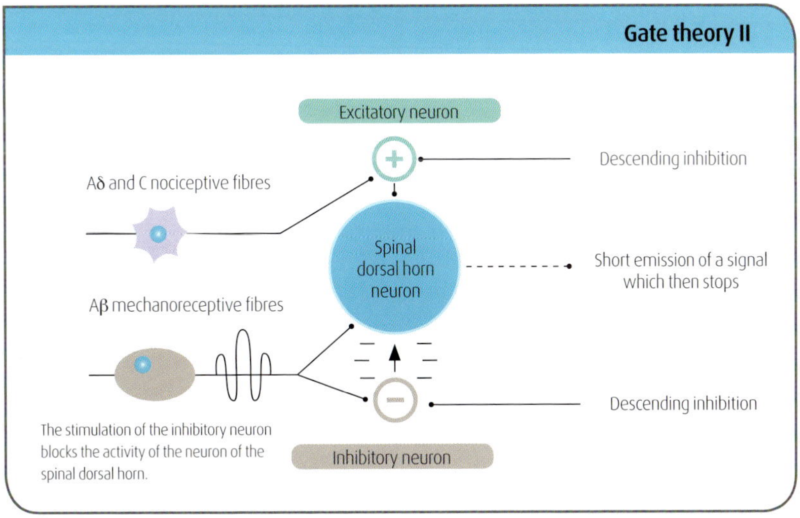

Let's take another example to understand this theory. All the readers have already experienced a sensation of relief when stroking a painful area. The gate control theory helps to explain why stroking the affected area, acupuncture or transcutaneous electrical stimulation have this analgesic effect. The three processes stimulate the Aβ receptors without stimulating the Aδ/C receptors. The inhibitory interneurons are therefore activated and send signals to the second-order neuron which receives information from the nociceptors (apart from the descending inhibitory information). This will cause the "closing of the gate" for signals sent from the nociceptive fibres to the second-order neuron, and as a consequence, the result will be an effect of relief and analgesia (fig. 4).

The effect that endogenous opiates have on pain perception also has other practical implications:

- Opioid analgesics and endogenous opioids produce their effect on the same receptors.
- An acute stress response favours the release of endogenous opioids, which would explain the temporary analgesia caused by such a response.
- Suckling could stimulate the release of endogenous opioids.
- The amniotic liquid could also stimulate the release of endogenous opioids. Placentophagy and licking the young could therefore contribute to the reduction of the pain caused by the delivery.

Neurotransmitters involved in nociception

There are both inhibitory (they hinder nociceptive signals) and excitatory (they facilitate nociception) transmitters (table 1).

The system of neurotransmitters involved in pain is very complex. One same neuron can be influenced by various neurotransmitters and, at the same time, release other neurotransmitters. It can also have many connections with other neurons which, in turn, possess numerous receptors for many different neurotransmitters.

The stress response associated with pain modifies the concentration, and therefore the activity, of these neurotransmitters. It is well-documented that chronic stress, which can be due to a state of chronic pain, reduces serotonin levels, one of the pain inhibitory neurotransmitters.

Table 1. Main excitatory and inhibitory neurotransmitters.

EXCITATORY NEUROTRANSMITTERS	Excitatory amino acids	Glutamate
		Aspartate
	Neuropeptides	P substance
		Neurotensin
		Vasoactive intestinal peptide
		Peptide related to the calcitonin gene
		Cholecystokinin
INHIBITORY NEUROTRANSMITTERS	GABA	
	Glycine	
	Serotonin	
	Dopamine	
	Noradrenaline	
	Acetylcholine	
	Histamine	
	Endorphines, enkephalins and dynorphins (released by the PAG)	

The reduction of the serotoninergic activity in the central nervous system has been linked to various behavioural changes in small animals, such as a greater tendency to show aggressiveness, be more impulsive when expressing this aggressiveness (with no, or very faint, previous warning signs), show ritualistic behaviours , etc. (which will be analysed in detail in the next chapters).

Sensitisation to pain

Once the pain pathways are stimulated, sensitivity to pain can be increased by new stimuli. This process is called sensitisation and includes two processes:

- **Hyperalgesia:** it is defined as an increase in the response to painful stimuli. That is to say, low-intensity painful stimuli give rise to an abnormally intense pain response.
- **Allodynia:** it could be defined as the process through which stimuli that are not normally painful cause pain.

Sensitisation (hyperalgesia and/or allodynia) can be explained through two general processes, peripheral and central sensitisation.

Peripheral sensitisation

It is also called primary hyperalgesia. Noxious stimuli are generally associated with inflammation of the damaged tissues. As a consequence of this inflammation, chemical mediators which attract inflammatory cells to the damaged area are released. These cells - macrophages, neutrophils, mastocytes and lymphocytes - release more mediators of inflammation. This inflammatory "soup" is formed by hydrogen and potassium ions, proteases, cyclooxygenase-2 (COX-2), prostaglandins, interleukins and cytokines, among many others. All these mediators will facilitate sensitisation by means of two phenomena:

- **Reduction of the excitation threshold of the Aδ/C receptors:** it should be remembered that they only respond to high-intensity stimuli, which can potentially cause tissue damage. As a consequence of this reduction, nociceptors will respond more intensively to painful stimuli (hyperalgesia) and will start to respond to stimuli that normally did not cause pain (allodynia).
- **Activation of silent nociceptors:** these receptors are formed by non-myelinated C fibres which, under normal conditions, do not respond to any stimuli. However, under the effects of the mediators of inflammation, they are activated and start discharging actively as a response to both noxious and innocuous stimuli. As a result, this will lead to both hyperalgesia and allodynia. Primary hyperalgesia corresponds to the area surrounding the damaged tissue.

Central sensitisation

It occurs because the neurons responsible for the transmission of pain modify their activity when they are bombarded with painful stimuli. As a consequence of this modification, when the same neurons are exposed to new noxious stimuli they will cause an exaggerated response. Central sensitisation causes secondary hyperalgesia, which affects areas located far from the tissue lesion.

Central sensitisation is a very complex process that is not known with accuracy. However, it seems to favour the tranmission of the stimulus and inhibit the endogenous pain modulation system (fig. 5).

It has been proposed that when the painful impulse reaches the spinal dorsal horn, it causes the release of neurotransmitters that facilitate subsequent depolarisations. More precisely, the main excitatory neurotransmitter,

Figure 5. Illustration of the central sensitisation process.

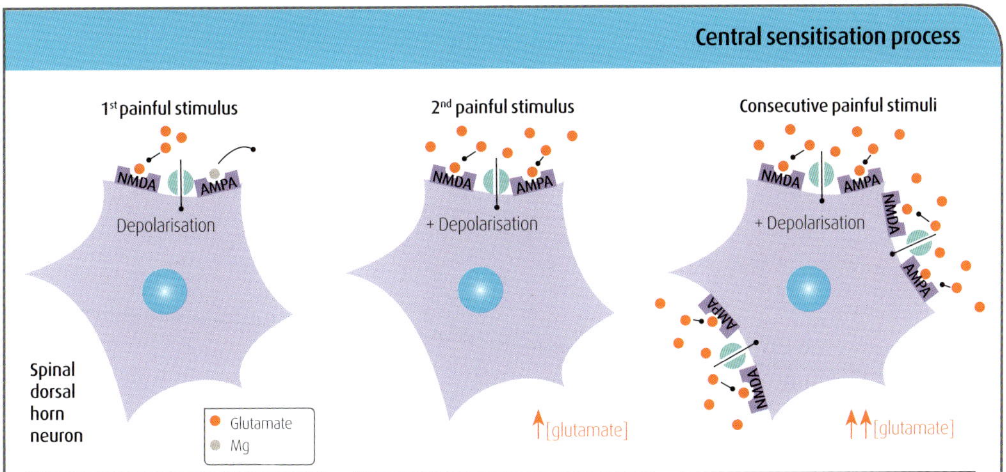

When the painful stimulus arrives, glutamate binds to the free NMDA receptors which causes neuronal depolarisation as well as the displacement of the Mg that occupied the AMPA receptors.

As the Mg has been displaced from the AMPA receptors, in the next painful stimulus, glutamate (whose concentration will have increased) will be able to bind to both NMDA and AMPA receptors and cause a greater depolarisation, therefore increasing the intensity of the stimulus and producing more pain.

There is an increase in the number of AMPA and NMDA receptors and in the glutamate concentration, which leads to a greater depolarisation, a more intense stimulus and therefore more pain.

glutamate, causes the depolarisation of neurons by binding to two receptors, AMPA (α-amino-3-hydroxy-5-methyl-4-isoxazolpropionic acid) and NMDA (N-methyl-D-aspartate) receptors.

When the first painful stimulus enters a neuron, glutamate is released. This latter binds easily to NMDA receptors, causing neuronal depolarisation, but not to AMPA receptors, since these are occupied by a magnesium ion. However, after the first stimulation, apart from binding to NMDA receptors, the released glutamate causes the displacement of the magnesium ion from the AMPA receptor. As a result, when a new stimulus reaches the neuron, glutamate will be able to bind to both AMPA and NMDA receptors, increasing depolarisation and therefore the intensity of the painful stimulus. In addition, the input of new action potentials will cause an increase in the number of AMPA and NMDA receptors in the neuronal membrane (up-regulation) that will facilitate neuronal conduction even more.

Central sensitisation can persist even once the initial cause of pain has been eliminated, which frequently contributes to the symptoms of chronic pain.

One of the objectives of veterinary practitioners, as regards diseases or complaints associated with pain, should be to prevent central sensitisation. A good analgesia should therefore always be provided before starting any procedures that may cause pain to the animal (e.g. pre, intra and post-surgical analgesia).

The exact duration of sensitisation to pain is not known. It could be expected to disappear along with inflammation, but the truth is that this is not usually the case. Its duration varies a lot and depends on the intensity, duration and nature of the painful stimulus, among other things.

Types of pain

Pain can be classified according to several criteria. The most common classifications are according to its origin and duration. As regards origin, pain can be somatic, visceral or neuropathic and as far as duration is concerned, pain can be acute or chronic.

Somatic pain

It occurs when there is a stimulation of the nociceptors of the skin, superficial muscles, joints, etc., which are abundant in these structures. They mainly respond to mechanical, chemical (also to mediators of inflammation) and thermal external stimuli. The pain they cause is easy to locate, which means that it is usually located at the site of the painful stimulus. If it radiates, it usually does so following the somatic nerve of the area. The pain is usually constant and rarely implies more general symptoms in humans (such as nausea). Some authors divide it into superficial somatic pain if it affects external structures (superficial skin and muscles) and deep somatic pain (deep muscles, tendons, periosteum or ligaments).

Visceral pain

This pain is caused by the activation of receptors located in the abdominal and thoracic organs. The nociceptors in these organs are less abundant and more scattered than somatic nociceptors. They mainly respond to ischaemia, distension and chemical stimuli (especially to mediators of inflammation). As opposed to somatic pain, visceral pain is diffuse and difficult to locate. The pain usually fluctuates in intensity with many peaks of intense pain. In humans, it is associated with nausea and vomitting. A characteristic of visceral pain is that, at least in humans, it causes referred pain, which is a pain that the central nervous system interprets as coming from a site other than where the lesion really is. The most accepted hypothesis to explain referred pain is that visceral nociceptors establish synapses in the same second-order neurons as some somatic nociceptors, so the CNS "believes" the stimulus comes from the surface of the body rather than from an organ.

Neuropathic pain

It is the pain caused by a lesion in the peripheral or central nervous system. It usually includes a central and peripheral sensitisation component (severe allodynia and hyperalgesia).The sensitisation occurring in neuropathic pain is due to various complex processes that take place at both peripheral and central levels, although only one of them (**neuromas**) will be detailed since the others go beyond the scope of this book. Neuropathic pain is thus partly due to the formation of neuromas, which are areas of intense nerve regeneration subsequent to a nerve lesion. Some of these neuromas cause ectopic discharges which are spontaneous and also respond to stimuli of a very low intensity. In addition, these neuromas (and other damaged fibres) develop new receptors, called **adrenergic receptors**, that will generate painful impulses when they are activated by the adrenaline released by the adjacent sympathetic nerves. This process is known as **sympathetic maintenance of pain** and will greatly contribute to neuropathic chronic pain.

A characteristic of neuropathic pain is that it does not respond well to treatment and, at least in humans, it is known for causing a fluctuating burning sensation, constant tingling, a sensation of electric shock, etc., combined with a

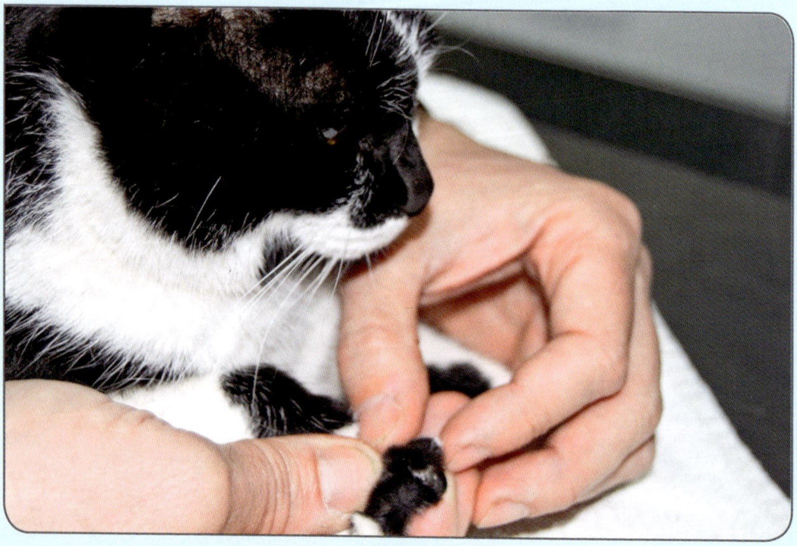

Figure 6. Declawed cat.

loss of sensitivity to heat. In animals, self-mutilation can be a sign of neuropathic pain and should be included in the differential diagnosis.

A special form of neuropathic pain is the pain occurring after the traumatic or surgical amputation of a limb, which is known in humans as the "phantom limb". The incidence in human medicine is not precisely known, but recent studies indicate that it could affect between 60 and 80% of the people who have suffered some kind of amputation. The pain is usually more frequent in the distal part of the phantom limb. Its intensity usually decreases with time. The evidence suggests that the animals that suffer an amputation (traumatic or surgical, such as tail-docking or ear-cropping) could also suffer from chronic neuropathic pain (figs. 6 and 7).

The effectiveness of the treatment, as in other forms of neuropathic pain, is limited. A study in human medicine suggests that the pre-surgical use of an epidural local anaeasthesic together with opioids reduces the incidence of post-surgical phantom limbs. However, other later studies could not reproduce the same findings.

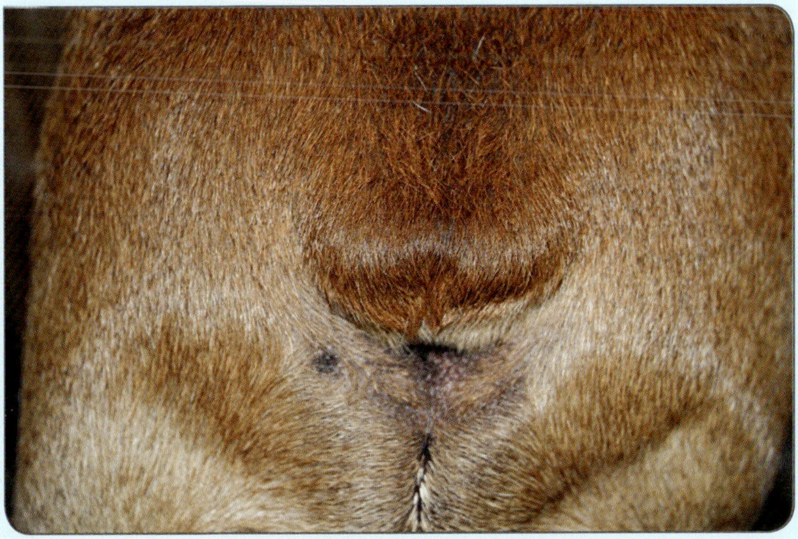

Figure 7. Tail docking in a dog.

Acute pain

Pain is also classified according to its duration. Acute pain is usually caused by tissue traumas. The intensity can be from moderate to severe and pain is usually most intense between 24-72 hours after the lesion. It is typically associated with an increase in the concentration of plasmatic glucocorticoids (fig. 8).

Chronic pain

Chronic pain is arbitrarily defined as a pain that lasts for more than 3-6 months. It includes an important component of sensitisation. Some examples of conditions causing chronic pain in animals are osteoarthritis (fig. 9), cancer or

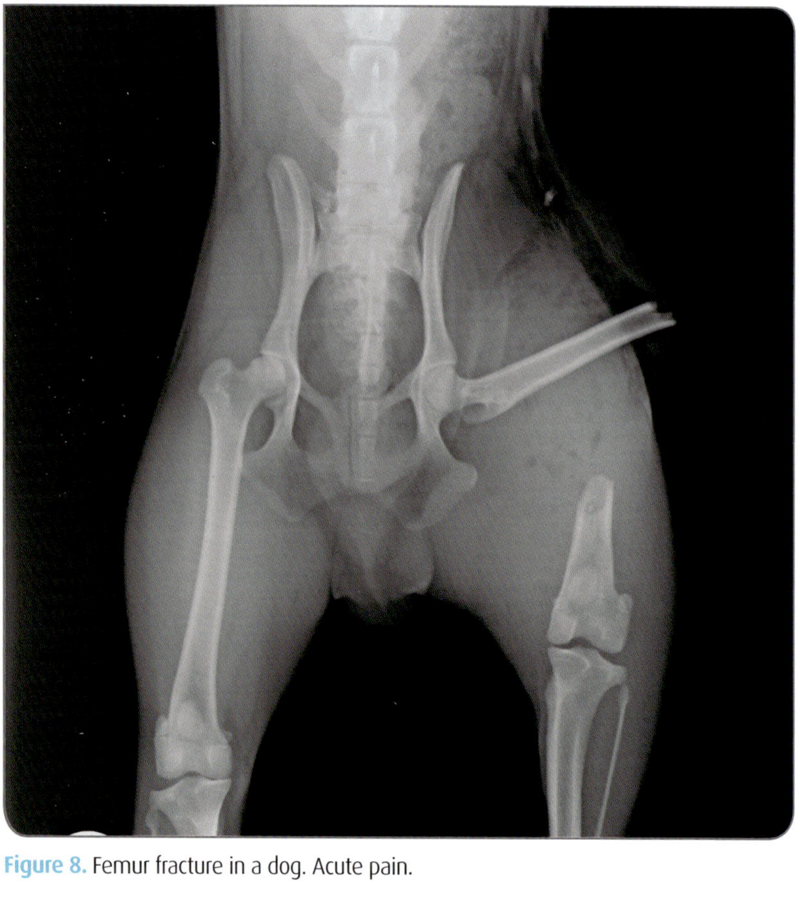

Figure 8. Femur fracture in a dog. Acute pain.

amputations. It is not usually associated with a plasmatic increase in glucocorticoids. The behavioural changes associated with chronic pain are usually more subtle than those caused by acute pain, but this does not mean that it is not a significant problem. It is in fact the opposite since, according to many authors, chronic pain is one of the main indicators of well-being in animals (this aspect will be detailed further on). Morever, there is evidence that chronic pain makes animals more sensitive to other acute stimuli. Some authors define chronic pain as pathologic pain.

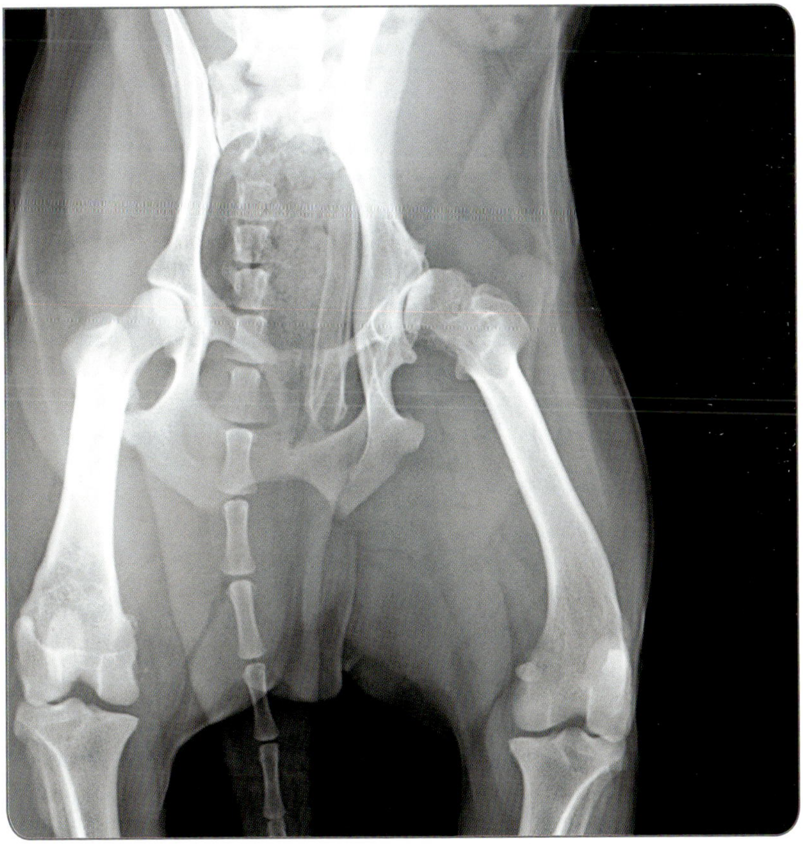

Figure 9. Signs of bone degeneration in a dog's hip. Chronic pain.

Pain in neonates

There are various widespread beliefs about pain in neonates among veterinary surgeons and many of them actually contradict each other. Some vets claim that neonates are not able to feel pain until after birth, and other theories point out that they can already feel it in the last stages of gestation. For example, the animal welfare laws of New Zealand protect mammal foetuses (Animal Welfare Act, 1999) after the first half of gestation and marsupials just after birth, when they still require a long development period in the marsupium. These laws were built on the assumption that these animals are already conscious and can therefore feel pain during these stages of development. On the other hand, some authors claim that neonates feel less pain than adults, while others think they feel more pain.

All these issues are of significant importance, especially when it comes to justifying the use of analgesics in painful procedures in newborn animals (e.g. cosmetic tail docking surgeries) or even its intrafoetal use (which is essential in human medicine and induced abortions). In short, two basic questions must be asked about pain neonates:

1. When do foetuses/newborns start to feel pain?
2. Is their sensitivity to pain the same as that of adults?

In order to answer these questions, the following elements must be taken into account:

- As seen at the beginning of this chapter, pain has a sensory component (nociception) and an emotional component (fig. 10), which implies conscious perception and causes the subjective and unpleasant feeling of pain. In other words, the consciousness of the animal is necessary for the feeling of pain to exist.
- Pain will therefore only be felt when the structures in charge of the conscious perception of pain are developed and functional.
- In a very simplified way, the structures in charge of the perception of pain are peripheral nociceptors, which are interneurons that form synapses with motor neurons (for nociception) or ascending pathways (to reach the brain

and allow the conscious perception of pain). The brain cortex, thalamus and thalamocortical fibres need to be functional for the emotional perception of pain.

Figure 10. Nerve structures involved in the spinal reflex and in pain perception via the spinothalamic tract.

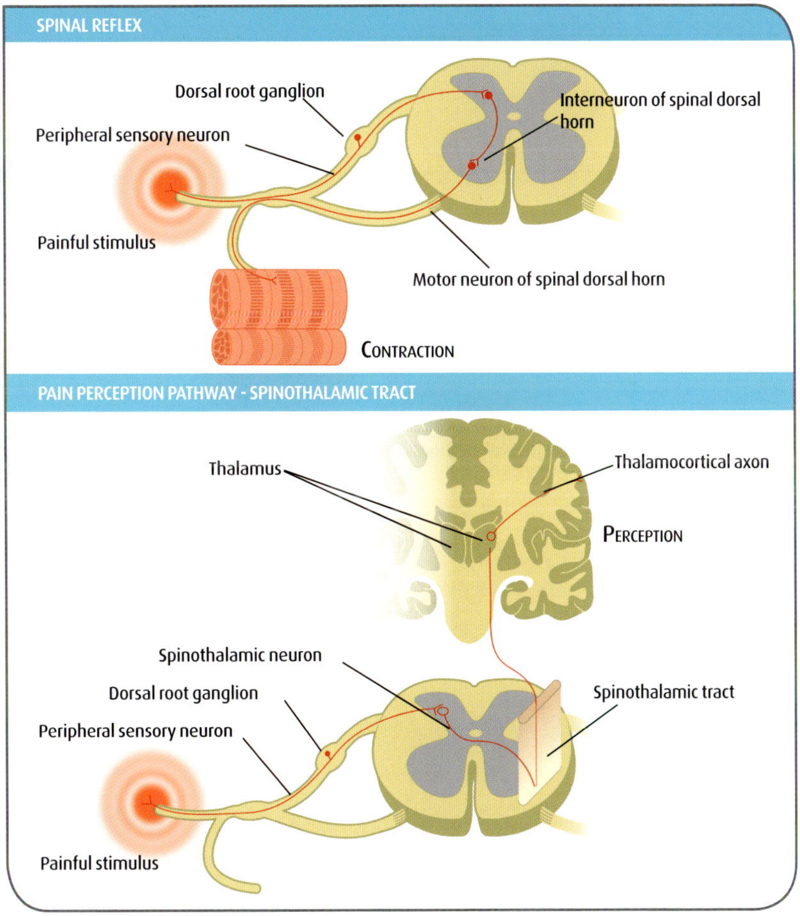

Extracted from: Lee S.J., Peter Ralston H.J., Drey E.A., Colin J., Rosen M.A. Fetal pain: A systematic multidisciplinary review of the evidence. *Journal of American Medical Association,* 2005; 294(8):947-954.

Neurological development

The development of the structures previously mentioned takes place at different times of the evolution of the foetus. The structures necessary for nociception develop at a very early stage. However, the structures in charge of the conscious perception of pain appear much later.

The general pattern of neurological development is quite similar among all the mammal species, independently from when the animal is born. Therefore, the fact that a specific species will start experiencing pain before, just after, or several days after birth will depend on the degree of maturation of the CNS at the moment of birth.

As previously said, the anatomical development of these structures is necessary but it is not sufficient to ensure conscious perception. They also need to be functional. In parallel with the changes in the electrical activity of the brain due to its maturation, changes in the behaviour of the individual can be observed. The start of the electrical activity in a specific area of the brain is therefore considered its functional start. The electrical activity is measured with an electroencephalogram (EEG).

In fact, during the maturation of any mammal's CNS, the electrical activity starts with initial sporadic peaks that evolve towards more sustained periods of activity, which turn first into an activity typical of sleep stages, although they are not differentiated, and then into well-differentiated REM (rapid eye movement) and non-REM stages. Finally, they become clearly differentiated cycles of sleep (with REM and non-REM stages) and wakefulness.

During the early stages of the CNS development, the short and sporadic electric potentials recorded in the brain cortex on the EEG do not allow conscious perception. All the recent studies consider the starting point of conscious perception to be when the first electric potentials that mark the differentiation between REM and non-REM stages are established, since it corresponds to the moment when the connections between subcortical structures and the brain cortex have been established and are functional.

In most mammals, this REM-non-REM differentiation does not take place until after birth. The most significant exception to this statement is probably the human species, in which the first evidence of thalamic input to subcortical and cortical areas can be observed, depending on the study, at week 20-22 and 23-24 of gestation respectively (anatomical evidence of development). In addition, the electrical activity indicating consciousness starts between weeks 29 and 30 of gestation.

SUMMARY

All mammals have a common pattern of neurological development. However, the stage of development at birth is different depending on the species and the ability to perceive pain will therefore appear before or after birth according to the state of development of each species at the time of birth.

Degree of maturation of the CNS at birth

Three large groups of mammal species can be distinguished according to the degree of maturation of the CNS at birth:

1. **Very immature species at birth:** joeys are exceptionally immature when they are born and most of their development takes place after birth in the marsupium. There is no evidence of electrical activity compatible with the perception of pain until after a third to half of the development period in the marsupium (e.g Wallabies -*Macropus eugenii eugenii*- spend an average 250 days in the marsupium).
2. **Moderately immature species at birth:** such as cats, dogs, mice, rats or rabbits. As for the previous group, REM and non-REM stages cannot be differentiated at birth, but this differentiation takes place between 3 and 14 days of life (a lot earlier than in the case of marsupials). It is therefore assumed that these species are not able to feel pain until this time has passed.
3. **Mature species at birth:** the most representative species in this group are lambs, foals, piglets, calves, baby guinea pigs and children. They have developed and functional structures for the perception of pain when they are born. In fact, in these species, the structures are completely mature after approximately 80% of the gestation.

However, various research lines support the theory that the conscious perception of pain in these species does not occur before birth, despite the fact that all the structures in charge are already functional at the end of gestation. There is a large amount of evidence that the maturation of cerebrocortical functionstakes place in a physiologically inhibitory environment, and that there are at least eight foetal, placental or uterine factors with an inhibitory effect on the EEG in the last half of gestation. Moreover, various studies have shown that neurologically mature foetuses do not respond to potentially painful stimuli until after birth. In other words, it has been observed that noxious stimuli are not able to change the sleep stage (REM or non-REM) to a state of consciousness in neurologically mature foetuses. However, the same stimuli do achieve it after birth. Other stimuli such as hypercapnia also alter the state of consciousness of the foetus in the last weeks of gestation. This is the clearest evidence of the inhibitory action of the gestation environment on the brain of the foetus in these species.

From a practical point of view, as far as dogs and cats are concerned, what has been seen so far could have important implications. In fact, neither the use of analgesics would be justified for painful procedures, nor the bans on surgical procedures with a cosmetic purpose (as it is the case with tail-docking in different autonomous communities in Spain, for example) provided that they are carried out just after birth. However, this is not the case. Painful experiences at a very early age, even though the animal does not perceive them at that time, can make the animal more sensitive. It seems that it could lead to a process of both central and peripheral long-term sensitisation. It has been observed that the tissue damaged during the postnatal period produces an overgrowth of nerve endings which causes the area to be hyper-innervated and hyper-sensitive. Furthermore, this exaggerated growth ocurrs in A and C fibres, but not in sympathetic fibres. In other words, the use of analgesics in painful conditions and procedures in neonates is necessary to avoid cases of hyperalgesia in the long-term.

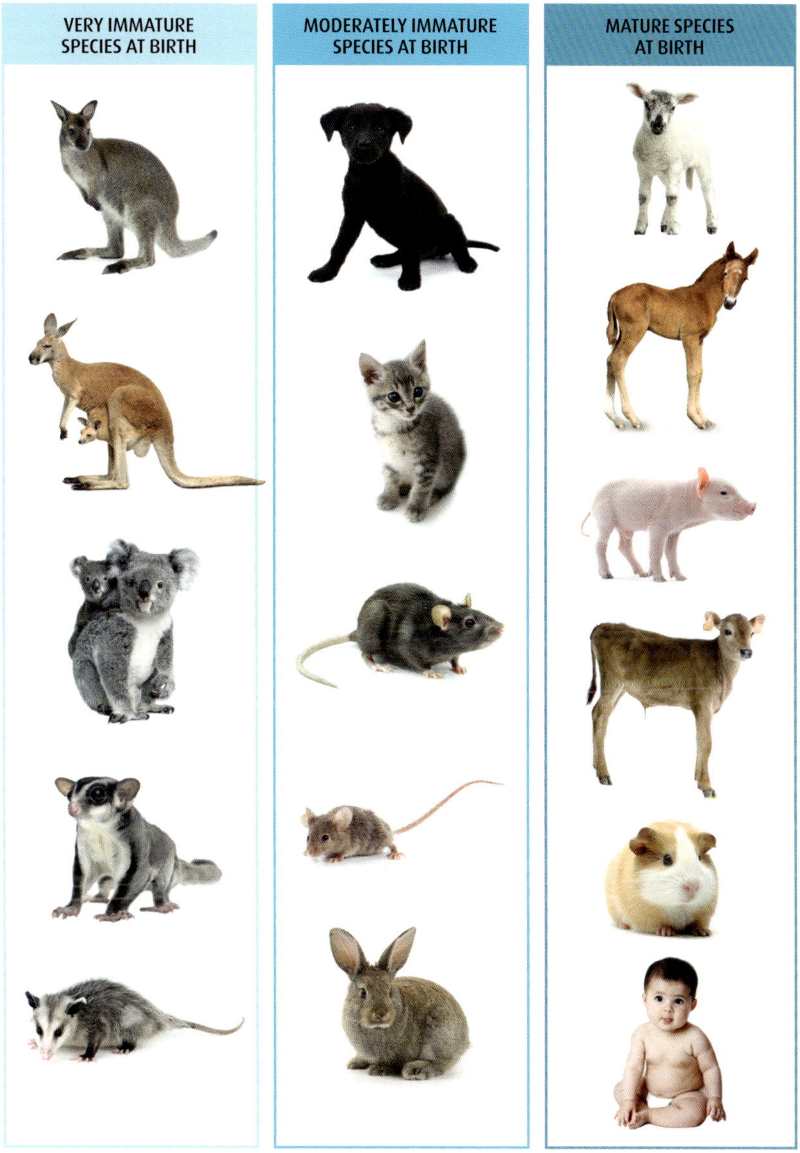
VERY IMMATURE SPECIES AT BIRTH
MODERATELY IMMATURE SPECIES AT BIRTH
MATURE SPECIES AT BIRTH

As regards whether neonates are more or less sensitive than an adult once conscious pain perception is present, there are disagreements too. Some studies point out that their response to pain is exaggerated, while others claim that they are less sensitive. Whatever the answer may be, from a clinical point of view, hyperalgesia and allodynia could occur in both cases, which is enough to justify the use of analgesia to treat pain in young animals.

KEY POINTS

The rigorous scientific study of foetal or neonatal pain shows difficulties as far as methodology and interpretation are concerned, which translates into numerous theories. The key points are:

1. Conscious pain perception cannot take place if the neurological structures responsible for it are not developed and functional.
2. This functional maturation occurs before or after birth depending on the species. In cats and dogs, it occurs a few days after birth (3-14 days).
3. However, this does not go against the use of analgesics in painful conditions and procedures since, although they do not perceive pain at that particular moment, it is known that both peripheral and central sensitisation occur, which triggers hyperlagesia and allodynia in the long term.
4. The use of analgesics in neonates who are suffering from pain or are about to undergo a painful surgical procedure is therefore necessary to the treatment.

Bibliography

Capner, C.A., Lascelles, B.D.X., Waterman-Pearson, A.E. Current British Attitudes to perioperative analgesia for cats and small mammals. *Veterinary Record*, 1999; 145:601-604.

Capner, C.A., Lascelles, B.D.X., Waterman-Pearson, A.E. Current British Attitudes to perioperative analgesia for dogs. *Veterinary Record*, 1999; 145:95-99.

Driessen, B., Zarucco, L. Pain: From diagnosis to efective treatment. *Clinical Techniques in Equine Practice*, 2007; 6(2):126-134.

Fecknell, P., Waterman-Pearson, A.E. *Pain Management in animals*. Editorial Saunders, Londres, 2000.

Grant, D. *Pain management in small animals a manual for veterinary nurses and technicians*. Editorial Elsevier, Edinburgh, 2006.

Gregory, N.G. Pain. In: *Physiology and behaviour of animal suffering*. Blackwell, 2004; 10:94-130.

Hellyer, P., Rodan, I., Downing, R., Hagedorn, J.E., Robertson, S.A. AAHA/AAFP Pain Management Guidelines for Dogs and Cats. *Journal of the American Hospital Association*, 2007; 43:235-248.

Lamont, L.A. Multimodal pain management in veterinary medicine: the physiologic basis of pharmacologic therapies. *Vet Clin Small Anim*, 2008; 38:1173-1186.

Lee, S.J., Peter Ralston, H.J., Drey, E.A., Colin, J., Rosen, M.A. Fetal pain: A systematic multidisciplinary review of the evidence. *Journal of American Medical Association*, 2005; 294(8):947-954.

Manteca, X. *Bienestar en vacuno de leche. Valoración y control del dolor.* Boehringer Ingelheim España, 2009.

Manteca, X. *Etología veterinaria*. Editorial Multimédica, Barcelona, 2009.

Mathews, K.A. Neuropathic pain in dogs and cats: If only they could tell us if they hurt. *Vet Clin Small Anim*, 2008; 38:1365-1414.

MELLOR, D.J., DIESCH, T.J. Onset of sentience: the potential for suffering in fetal and newborn farm animals. *Applied Animal Behaviour Science*, 2006; 100:48-57.

MELLOR, D.J., DIESCH, T.J., JOHNSON, C.B. Legal and animal welfare implications of when conciousness first appears in developing young and of the potential for delayed onset of increased pain sensitivity. Australian Animal Welfare Strategy-AAWS International animal welfare conference, 2010.

MELLOR, D.J., GREGORY, N.G. Responsiveness, behavioural arousal and awareness in fetal and newborn lambs: experimental, practical and therapeutic implications. *New Zeland Veterinary Journal*, 2003; 51:2-13.

PATTISON, D., FITZGERALD, M. The neurobiology of infant pain: development of excitatory and inhibitory neurotransmission in the spinal dorsal horn. *Regional Anesthesia and Pain Medicine*, 2004; 29(1):36-44.

ROBERTSON, S.A. What is pain? *J Am Vet Med Assoc*, 2002; 221(2):202-205.

2

IDENTIFICATION, CAUSES AND TREATMENT OF PAIN IN COMPANION ANIMALS

Classification of pain

There are various ways of classifying pain (table 1), for instance, according to its duration, cause, intensity, etc. However, it should be taken into account that pain can be multifactorial and that, in addition, it can be modified by the evolution of the disease itself (it is not a static process) or by the treatment administered. That is why a more up-to-date classification (table 2) would divide pain into:

- **Adaptive** (the pain has a protective function).
- **Non adaptive** (when adaptive pain is not treated correctly and physical changes take place in the central nervous system).

Non adaptive pain is more difficult to treat. It occasionally requires more specific drugs such as NMDA receptor antagonists (see chapter General concepts and physiology of pain) like amantadine and gabapentin to restore central transmission.

Table 1. Types of pain, general classification.

CLASSIFICATION	PRESENTATION	CHARACTERISTIC	EXAMPLE
According to its duration	Acute	Lasts less than 2 weeks.	Tooth pain.
	Chronic	Lasts more than 3 months.	Cancer pain.
According to its pathogeny	Neuropathic	Caused by of a lesion of the nervous system.	Spinal lesion.
	Nociceptive	Caused by the stimulation of pain receptors.	Sharp pain.
	Inflammatory	Caused by tissue damage and inflammation.	Postoperative pain.
According to its location	Visceral	Activation of internal pelvic, abdominal or thoracic visceral nociceptors.	Hepatic lesion.
	Somatic	Activation of skin, bone and soft tissue nociceptors.	Arthritis.
According to its course	Intermittent	Episodes of pain followed by pain-free periods.	
	Continuous	Always present.	
According to its intensity	Mild	A daily routine can be carried out.	Muscular lesion.
	Moderate	Interferes with daily routine.	Post-surgery recovery.
	Severe	Interferes with rest.	Spinal disc herniation.

Table 2. Types of pain, current classification.

TYPE OF PAIN	DEFINITION	CLASSIFICATION
ADAPTIVE PAIN	Pain that appears as a result of the normal response of the damaged tissue.	Inflammatory. Nociceptive.
NON-ADAPTIVE PAIN	Pain caused by a lesion of the nervous system.	Neuropathic. Functional. Central.

Identification of the signs of pain

Physiological and behavioural changes occur as a consequence of pain. Some of the physiological changes that take place, such as an increase in cortisol for example, trigger a stress response, which can in turn have very negative consequences on the animal when it is chronic.

Therefore, it is paramount to learn how to identify the signs that indicate that an animal is in pain. However, there is not a standard way of assessing pain, as there are differences between species and even within the same species.

In the feline and canine species, the observation of the animal's behaviour is the best way of identifying whether it is in pain or not. That is why it is important to take the peculiarities of each species and each animal into consideration.

It is very important to differentiate pain from dysphoria (aberrant behaviour) and other stress signs (e.g. fear). When animals present with pain, it is possible, except when it is very acute, to distract and calm them temporarily by means of an interaction. However, when they are suffering from dysphoria, interactions do not manage to stop the animal's behaviour. In this case, the reaction can be due to the paradoxical effect of some of the analgesic drugs administered (e.g. opioids) or to the general anaesthesia. The administration of a sedative or an antagonist will allow this paradoxical effect to be reversed in the patients that present with this reaction.

Individual differences in the expression of pain

Differences are not only observed between species. Two individuals of the same species can express pain in a very different way. This can be due to different factors. Some of the factors to take into consideration are:

Age

Young animals, in particular neonates, are more sensitive to pain.

Genetics

Some authors suggest that certain breeds that are used more for work (Labrador Retriever, German Shepherd) could express pain in a less obvious manner than other breeds, such as toy breeds for example.

Sex

Differences between the two sexes have been observed in humans (in both directions) according to the pain stimulus.

Previous experiences

After a manipulation that has turned out to be painful, the animal can react in a more intense way -due to the anxiety of facing the same painful stimulus- if it experiences or expects the same manipulation again.

Temperament

The animal's temperament can also have an influence on the response. This aspect will be dealt with in the next chapter.

Behavioural changes

When an animal presents with pain, the most characteristic sign is a change in its behaviour. Depending on whether the pain is acute, persistent or chronic, the changes in behaviour observed will be different. The changes most commonly observed in the canine and feline species are described in tables 3, 4 and 5.

Table 3. Behavioural changes which may be observed and that are associated with pain in dogs.

TYPE OF PAIN	CHANGE OBSERVED
Acute pain/wound	Slight shivering. Attempt to hide behind the owner. Attempt to escape from the consultation room. Vocalisations and aggressiveness (associated with intense pain).
Persistent/postoperative pain	Whining. Changes of position (the dog is reluctant to sit or lie down, arches its back). Is reluctant to move. Loss of appetite. Changes in facial expression. Depending on the affected area: ear shaking in cases of ear pain, blepharospasm in cases of eye pain, salivation in cases of mouth pain... Friendly interactions with staff are reduced. Licks, bites or touches the affected area with its paw. Apathy or aggressiveness can appear. Fast and superficial respiration (intense abdominal pain).
Chronic pain	Reduced activity. Muscular stiffness. Muscular atrophy and uneven claw wear when the chronic pain affects one limb. Arched spine with forelimb loading when there is bilateral hip or lower spine pain.

Table 4. Behavioural changes which may appear and that are associated to pain in cats.

TYPE OF PAIN	CHANGE OBSERVED
Acute pain/wound	Shivering. Slight growling. Marked aggressiveness. Attempt to escape.
Persistent/postoperative pain	The cat is depressed, silent and tense and does not move. Tries to hide and does not respond to stroking. Prefers to remain in sternal decubitus position and can react aggressively when manipulated in the postoperative period. Vocalisations are rare. Shows changes in facial expression. Rubs, licks or bites the affected area.
Chronic pain	Reduced activity (plays and goes outside less, more time sleeping). Loss of appetite (weight loss). Inappropriate elimination (incorrect use of the litter tray). Less grooming (unhealthy hair coat). Chronic pain in one limb may take the form of a limp or muscular atrophy.

In general, it can be said that:

Acute pain/wound	⇨	Avoidance and escape behaviour.
Persistent /postoperative	⇨	Vigilance and protective behaviour.
Chronic	⇨	Depression, inhibited behaviour.

Table 5. Most common physiological and behavioural changes in an indivudal showing pain.

GENERAL SIGNS	SPECIFIC SIGNS
Loss of normal behaviour	Reduced activity. Lethargy. Loss of appetite. Less grooming (cats). More complicated habdling in hospital.
Expression of abnormal behaviours	Inappropriate elimination. Vocalisation. Aggressiveness. Reduced interaction with other family members. Altered facial expression. Altered posture. Restlessness. Hiding (especially cats).
Reaction to manipulation	Increased body tension. Shivering in response to palpation of the affected area.
Physiological parameters	Increase in heart rate. Increase in respiratory rate. Increase in temperature. Increase in blood pressure. Dilated pupils.

How to measure pain

The scale/system used to assess pain must be validated (the scale must really assess pain), highly sensitive (able to detect slight differences in pain intensity) dolor) and highly reliable (same score when the scale is applied to several individuals with a similar pain or when it is used by different people; repeatability).

Ther are many scales to measure pain. Some are only based on behavioural parameters, while others combine the assessment of behavioural and physiological parameters (table 6).

Table 6. Pain assessment scales.

SCALE USED	PARAMETERS OBSERVED
Simple descriptive scale (SDS)	Behavioural.
Visual analogue scale (VAS)	Behavioural.
Dynamic and interactive analogue visual scale (DIVAS)	Behavioural.
Variable rating scale (VRS) (University of Melbourne scale)	Behavioural and physiological.
Descriptive pain assessment scale	Behavioural and physiological.
Glasgow pain scale	Behavioural.

Simple descriptive scales

There are several examples of simple descriptive scales. The observer must choose between 3-5 options after observing and manipulating the patient (see examples in tables 7 and 8).

Table 7. Simple descriptive scale used in cats.

SCORE	CRITERIA
0	No signs of pain.
1	The cat is content, friendly and purrs. Tenses up if pressure is applied on the wound but not when stroking the affected area.
2	The cat is content and tenses up if the affected area is stroked.
3	The cat seems uncomfortable but the wound can be touched.
4	The cat seems uncomfortable and does not let the wound be touched. Can growl and hiss.

Table 8. Simple descriptive scale used in dogs.

OBSERVATION	SCORE	CRITERIA
Vocalisation	0	Does not vocalise.
	1	Vocalisations are reduced if the animal is talked to with a soft tone and stroked.
	2	Vocalisations are not reduced with a soft tone or stroking.
Movements	0	None.
	1	Frequent changes of position.
	2	Thrashing.
Restlessness	0	Asleep or calm.
	1	Slight restlessness.
	2	Moderate restlessness.
	3	Severe restlessness.

The advantage of this type of scales is that they are easy to use, but they have the disadvantage of being very subjective as well as of poor reliability and sensitivity.

Visual analogue scale (VAS)

If this scale is used, the observer must place a mark on a 100 mm line to indicate the intensity of pain observed in the patient.

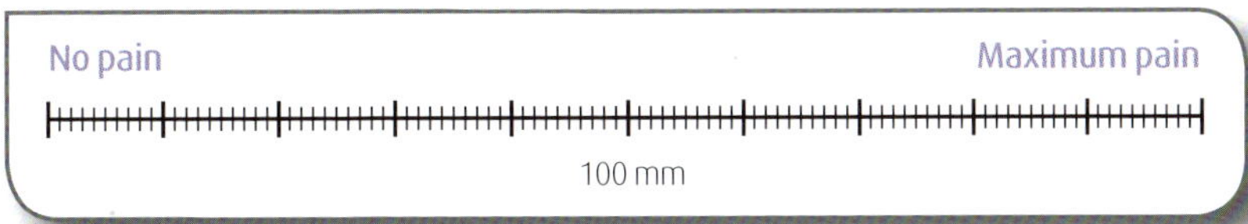

Disadvantages:

- The assessment could be influenced by the observer's visual and locomotor coordination (if the observer suffered from an ocular or motor disorder, this could result in a less precise measurement and a mistake of up to 7 mm).
- Low reliability if the observers are not very experienced.

Dynamic and interactive analogue visual scale (DIVAS)

This scale is a modification of the visual analogue scale. Apart from observing the patient, the examiner must assess its reactions when the painful area is approached, touched or manipulated.

Advantages: both the VAS and the DIVAS are more sensitive than the simple descriptive scale.

Variable rating scales

With these scales, the observer assesses physiological parameters in addition to watching the animal's behaviour.

The scale used at the University of Colorado to measure acute pain in dogs and cats and that developed by the University of Melbourne (tables 9 and 10) are two examples of this type of scales. The University of Melbourne scale is divided into 6 categories (physiological data, response to palpation, activity, mental status, posture and vocalisations). Each category is divided into different levels to which a number is assigned.

Table 9. University of Melbourne pain scale.

CATEGORY		DESCRIPTOR	SCORE
Physiologic data	a	Within reference range.	0
	b	Dilated pupils.	2
	c. Choose only one option (in relation to pre-operative rate).	% increase in heart rate: > 20% > 50% > 100%	 1 2 3
	d. Choose only one option (in relation to pre-operative rate).	% increase in respiratory rate: > 20% > 50% > 100%	 1 2 3
	e	Hyperthermy.	1
	f	Salivation.	2
Response to palpation	Choose only one option.	No change from preoperative behaviour.	0
		Guards or reacts when touched (turns head to affected area, tenses up, protection posture).	2
		Guards or reacts before being touched	3
Activity	Choose only one option.	At rest: Sleeping. Semiconscious. Awake.	 0 0 1
		Eats.	0
		Restless (pacing continuously, getting up and down).	2
		Rolling/thrashing.	3
Mental status	Choose only one option.	Submissive.	0
		Overtly friendly.	1
		Wary.	2
		Aggressive.	3
Posture	a	Guards and protects the affected area.	2
	b. Choose only one option.	Lateral recumbency.	0
		Sternal recumbency.	1
		Sitting or standing, head up.	1
		Standing, head hanging down.	2
		Moving.	1
		Abnormal posture.	2
Vocalisations	Choose only one option.	No vocalising.	0
		Vocalises when touched.	2
		Intermittent vocalisation.	2
		Continuous vocalisation.	3

Table 10. Feline acute pain scale.

Pain scale	EXAMPLE	PHYSIOLOGICAL AND BEHAVIOURAL PARAMETERS	RESPONSE TO PALPATION	BODY TENSION
0	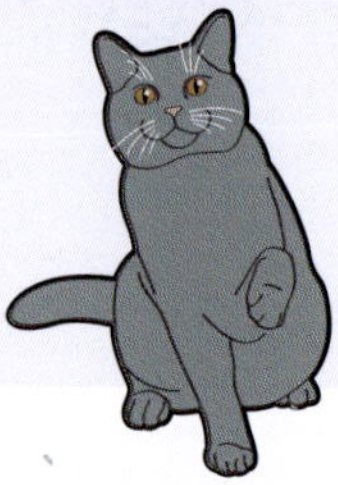	☐ Content and quiet when unattended. ☐ Comfortable when resting. ☐ Interested in or curious about surroundings.	☐ Not bothered by palpation of wound or surgery site, or by palpation elsewhere.	Minimal.
1	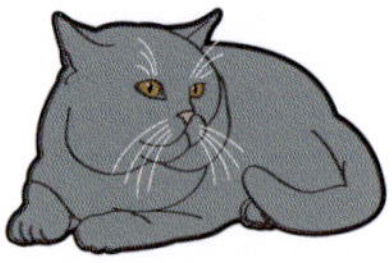	☐ Signs are often subtle and not easily detected in the hospital setting. ☐ Earlier signs at home may be withdrawal from surroundings or change in normal routine. ☐ In the hospital, may be content our slightly unsettled. ☐ Less interested in surroundings but will look around to see what is going on.	☐ May or may not react to palpation of wound or surgery site.	Mild.
2	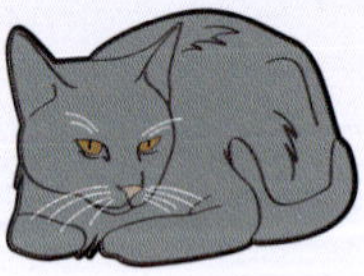	☐ Decreased responsiveness, seeks solitude. ☐ Lies curled up or sits tucked up with eyes partially or mostly closed. ☐ Hair coat appears rough. ☐ May intensively groom an area that is painful or irritating. ☐ Decreased appetite, not interested in food.	☐ Responds aggressively or tries to escape if painful area is palpated or approached. ☐ Tolerates attention, may even perk up when petted.	Mild to moderate. **Reassess analgesic plan.**
3	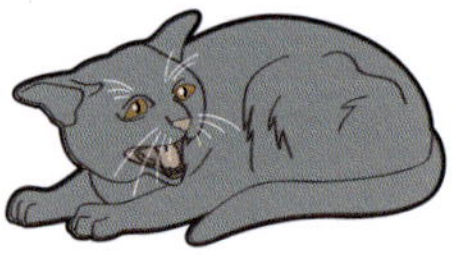	☐ Constantly yowling, growling or hissing when unattended. ☐ May bite or chew at wound, but unlikey to move if left alone.	☐ Growls or hisses at non-painful palpation. ☐ Reacts aggressively to palpation, adamantly pulls away to avoid any contact.	Moderate. **Reassess analgesic plan.**
4	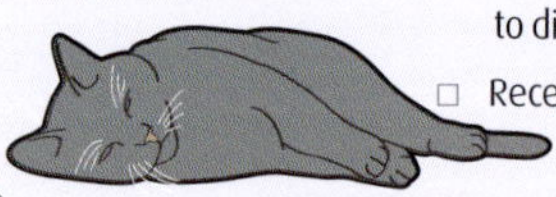	☐ Prostrate. ☐ Potentially unresponsive to or unaware or surroundings, difficult to distract from pain. ☐ Receptive to care.	☐ May not respond to palpation. ☐ May be rigid to avoid painful movement.	Moderate to severe. **Reassess analgesic plan.**

Modified from Hellyer, P.W., Uhrig, S.R., Robinson, N.G. Feline Acute Pain Scale, Colorado State University, Veterinary Medical Center, 2006.

Causes of pain

Various correlations between the intensity/duration of the pain and certain signs or findings derived from the disease have been observed in humans. For example, there is a positive correlation between the pro-inflammatory prostaglandin PGE_2 levels in synovial liquid and pain intensity in patients with arthritis. It is known that the processes that include picking up the painful stimuli, their transmission and modulation are very similar between the human species and animals. This information from human medicine (table 11) can therefore be of great use in veterinary medicine. First of all, it can help the veterinary surgeon to decide on which analgesia protocol to follow. For instance, when deciding which analgesia to administer in animals with cancer, the size of the tumour and its probable innervation are more relevant that the number of tumours itself. Secondly, it provides information about what diseases and complaints can be painful. For example, in cases of femoral head necrosis, a collapse of the hip joint can be a good indicator of pain. Thirdly, it creates a pathway to research on parameters that can be reliable indicators of pain in certain diseases in animals. For example, in animals used in sports competitions, creatine kinase can be a good indicator of myalgia in addition to its common use as an indicator of a muscle lesion or a lesion due to effort.

Table 11. Examples of pathological findings quantitatively related to the intensity or duration of pain in humans.

PATHOLOGY	FINDINGS CORRELATED WITH PAIN
Inflammation	Rash. Oedema. Erythema.
Pancreatitis	Infiltration of immune cells at perineural level. GAP-43 in nerve fibres.
Ileitis	Length of affected intestine.
Synovitis	Effusion. Plasmatic and synovial levels of monocyte chemoattractant protein 1 (MCP-1).
Arthritis	Inflammatory prostaglandin PGE_2 levels in synovial fluid. Fat deposits in muscles.
Back pain	Sclerosis. Spinal stenosis. Osteophytes. Substance P levels in the CSF.
Spinal disc herniation	IL-8 in the CSF.
Myalgias	Serum creatine kinase. Muscle oedema.
Tumours	Size of tumour in pancreatic, skin, intestinal, hepatic, biliary duct and cauda equina tumours. Invasion of an organ by nerve fibres.
Dermal ulcers	Size of the ulcer.
Mastodynias	Size of the mammary duct.
Neuropathies	Reduced density of intraepidermal nerve fibres.
Endometriosis	Size of the ovarian endometrioma. Extension of the adhesions.
Hepatopathies	Portal fibrosis.
Tooth pain	Chronic pulp disease. Saliva electrolyte levels. Swelling.

Modified from Gregory, N.G., *Animal Welfare*, 2010, 19:437-448.

The most common causes of pain in the dog and cat can be grouped into four categories: routine procedures, diseases and lesions, surgery and labour.

Routine procedures

Any procedure or manipulation of the animal (vaccines, X-rays, sampling, ultrasound scans, etc.), although carried out in a gentle manner, can be painful and/or increase discomfort in an animal in pain.

We can try to minimise pain and/or stress by adopting a series of measures:

- Our work must be carried out in a comfortable and quiet place. Working in areas where people are continuously coming in or where vocalisations of other animals can be heard should be avoided.
- The animal must be held properly. The veterinary surgeon and the nurse must know how to hold the animal so that they do not cause pain during manipulation. On occasions, a gentle restraint is preferable (especially in cats) to prevent the animal from getting more nervous. At other times, a towel can be used to hold the cat. Depending upon the procedure and if the state of the animal allows it, distractions and rewards can be used during manipulation. The objective is to reduce the probability of the animal reacting with fear and/or aggressively as much as possible.
- If a catheter needs to be placed, a local or topical anaesthetic can be applied on the shaved skin a few minutes before the procedure.
- For certain manipulations, such as ear cleaning/exploration of an animal with otitis, or anal sacs emptying, an opioid can be administered. These analgesic drugs allow pain to be reduced and help preventing the appearance of fear/anxiety problems derived from these manipulations.

Diseases and lesions

One of the most common clinical signs, which is present in many diseases and certain lesions, is inflammation. Inflammation if the most frequent cause of pain. It must be remembered that, apart from the pain directly derived from it, inflammation produces hyperalgesia and allodynia (see previous chapter).

The association between pain and certain diseases and/or lesions (a fracture for example) is unquestionable. However, there are many other causes of pain that we do not take into account or simply underestimate. For example, when an animal has a bone tissue tumour, a treatment with analgesic drugs is more likely to be considered if the tumour is located in soft tissue. It is therefore important to be familiarised with all the pahologies and lesions that can be associated with pain.

Surgeries

According to the type of surgery, post-surgical pain is more or less intense (table 12). It is important to know the intensity of pain associated to a specific surgery in order to choose the most appropriate analgesia protocol. Once the surgery is over, it is recommended to monitor the animal at least every 30 minutes to ensure that the patient is not in pain or does not suffer from other complications derived from the operation. This is better done by the same person.

When the procedure is expected to cause intense pain (thoracotomy, abdominal, orthopaedic or spinal surgery), it is recommended to use powerful opiates during pre-surgery. The drug will be chosen depending on the estimated duration of the operation. In addition, the administration of an analgesic drug immediately before surgery will allow a reduction in the amount of anaesthetics required (see Appendix I). Amputations are also considered operations with intense post-surgical pain. On occasions, the phantom limb syndrome can appear after the amputation. This is due to a spontaneous regeneration of the area (also known as neuroma) that entails peripheral sensitisation and, therefore, chronic pain. In humans, 60% of the patients that have undergone an amputation experience phantom limb syndrome. An interesting fact is that, on occasions, the pain can appear even a year after the operation.

Table 12. Intensity of pain caused by different types of procedures in the dog.

PROCEDURE	PRESENCE OR ABSENCE OF PAIN
Taking off stitches. Nail clipping.	No pain
Suturing. Placement of a urinary catheter. Dental cleaning. Ear exploration and cleaning.	Mild pain
Ovariohysterectomy. Castration. Cesarean section. Tooth extraction.	Moderate pain
Thoracotomy. Laparotomy. Laminectomy. Amputation. Eye surgery.	Intense pain

Modified from Stafford, K., *The welfare of dogs.* Ed. Springer, Dordrecht, The Netherlands, 2007.

The formation of neuromas after tail docking, a very common practice in certain dog breeds (e.g. the English Cocker Spaniel) for purely aesthetic purposes, has been shown, which suggests that the same may happen after other mutilations. Ear cropping is another example of an amputation for aesthetic reasons that can cause very intense post-surgical pain. Some authors recommend using epidural analgesia before surgery and a local aneasthetic after it, although the response is very variable.

In the feline species, declawing is still relatively common to prevent the cat from scratching furniture. This practice is very painful since it involves amputating not only the claw, but also the first phalange. On top of that, it must be added that we deprive the cat of one of the forms of marking it most uses to communicate. In most cases, inappropriate marking (on sofas, curtains) could be avoided by placing a scratcher in an appropriate place.

Labour

Although females endure pain better during labour (their pain threshold is higher due to the secretion of endogen opioids), both uterine contractions and cervical dilation cause pain. Some authors claim that induced labour is more painful than spontaneous labour.

Treatment of pain

There are several options, which are not exclusive, to treat pain. The measures detailed next are not mutually exclusive and are actually much more effective when combined.

1. Administering drugs with analgesic properties.
2. Improving handling and housing conditions.
3. Feeding nutraceuticals.
4. Using alternative therapies (acupuncture).

Drug treatment

There are many drugs that can provide analgesia (table 13). However, before administering an analgesic, we should consider the following elements:

- Whether the procedure we are about to carry out is painful.
- The area we want to treat (table 14).
- Whether the animal also presents with behavioural problems, such as fear or anxiety, that can worsen the pain derived from the procedure we are about to carry out.
- Whether there is any medication contraindicated for this patient (chronic diseases, adverse reactions to certain drugs, current state of health, characteristics of the species regarding the metabolism of certain drugs, etc.). For instance, the use of certain drugs should be avoided in the feline species since it is known that a poor glucuronidation, due to a lower availability of isoforms of the hepatic enzyme UDP-glucuronosyltransferase (involved in the second phase of metabolisation), causes cats to be more prone to adverse reactions if they are administered phenolic drugs (paracetamol) or drugs with an elevated half-life such as carprofen or salicylates (aspirin).

Table 13. Most used drugs for the treatment of pain.

DRUGS	PROPERTIES
Opioids	Analgesic, allow a reduction in the amount of anaesthetic required.
NSAIDs	Analgesic, anti-inflammatory and antipyretic.
Local anaesthetics	Analgesic, allow a reduction in the amount of anaesthetic required.
α_2-agonists	Analgesic, sedative and muscle relaxant.
NMDA inhibitors (ketamine, amantadine)	Provide some analgesia.
Psychopharmaceuticals (amitriptyline, clomipramine)	Provide some analgesia, anxiolytic.
Anticonvulsants (gabapentin)	Provide some analgesia, sedation and muscle relaxation.
Tramadol	Provides some analgesia.

Table 14. Site of action of analgesic drugs.

SITE OF ACTION	DRUGS
Drugs acting at peripheral nociceptors.	• Local anaesthetics.
Drugs acting at primary afferent fibres.	• Local anaesthetics. • α_2-agonists.
Drugs acting at the dorsal horn.	• Opioids. • NSAIDs. • α_2-agonists. • Local anaesthetics.
Drugs acting at thalamocortical structures.	• Opioids. • α_2-agonists.
Drugs acting at descending antinociceptive pathways.	• Opioids. • α_2-agonists.
Drugs minimising development of or showing efficacy during peripheral sensitisation.	• Opioids. • NSAIDs.
Drugs minimising development of or showing efficacy during central sensitisation.	• Ketamine. • Amantadine. • Gabapentin. • COX-2-specific NSAIDs.

Modified from Leight A. Lamont, Multimodal pain management in veterinary medicine: the physiologic basis of pharmacologic therapies. *Vet Clin Small Anim*, 2008; 38.

Opioids (narcotics)

General considerations

Considered the most analgesic drugs. Very effective to treat acute pain. They bind with the opioid receptors, thus blocking the transmission of nociceptive signals at both central and peripheral levels. Depending on the affinity of the drug for the receptor and which receptor it binds to (mu, kappa or delta), opioids produce sedation and euphoria in addition to analgesia. The most powerful opiates (morphine, pethidine, fentanyl) are usually less effective in cats.

They can be used before any surgical intervention to reduce the amount of anaesthetics. In general, they have a short-term effect (from 15 minutes to 8 hours depending on the drug).

Their effects are reversible by administering an antagonist such as naloxone or naltrexone.

Most common side effects

- Buprenorphine and butorphanol can cause behavioural alterations in healthy cats and dogs if they are not administered along with a sedative.
- Cardiovascular: bradychardia (morphine and fentanyl). They must be injected slowly to avoid hypotension if administered intravenously.
- Respiratory depression.
- Urinary retention in prolonged administration.
- Hyperthermy in cats. This is not observed with the administration of buprenorphine and butorphanol.
- Gastrointestinal: nauseas, vomiting and salivation after the administration of morphine and hydromorphone. The combined administration with acepromazine reduces this effect. Also intestinal stasis, which occasionally causes constipation.
- Marked mydriasis in cats: this may cause them to bump into objects and not see us approaching correctly. As a result, they may react aggressively and/or with fear.
- Behavioural alterations: euphoria, purring, rolling skin syndrome and pedaling movements of forelimbs. Dysphoria (due to the activity of the kappa receptor) has been observed in this species after the administration of butorphanol. It seems to be related to high doses of the drug.

Drug interactions

The combined use of opioids (fentanyl) and monoamine oxidase inhibitors (selegiline, amitraz) should be avoided. Pyrexia, coma, stiffness, hypertension, seizures and delirium have been described in humans. Although no studies have been conducted on animals, it is preferable to use morphine if an opioid drug needs to be administered to a patient treated with an MAOI (monoamine oxidase inhibitor).

Most used opioid drugs

- **Meperidine:** this drug is not as powerful as morphine. However, it is less sedative and causes less vomiting. IV administration is associated to excitement and IM administration is therefore advised. Its effects appear very quickly, about 10-15 minutes after administration and the duration of the analgesia varies between 1 and 2 hours. Its structure, similar to that of atropine, gives it an anticholinergic effect. This antispasmodic activity turns it into the only opioid that can be administered in cases of pancreatitis or biliary disease.
- **Fentanyl:** its effects appear very quickly, approximately 2-5 minutes after IV administration. The duration of the analgesia is very short, from 5 to 20 minutes. If it is administered by infusion, this should be done over two hours to avoid any toxic effect due to its accumulation in the organism. Transdermal patches are very useful to treat pain in cats, although no studies about its efficacy on chronic pain in this species have been conducted. In critical patients, hypothermy, hypovolemia, and a diminished skin perfusion can reduce its absorption. During its absorption, administering other opioids (except butorphanol) is recommended to treat pain, since the therapeutic levels are reached 24 hours after placing the patch. Its effects are maintained for at least 72 hours.
- **Morphine:** drug of choice in cases of intense pain. More effective on dogs than on cats. This can be due to cats' lower ability to produce active metabolites of morphine. It can be administered IV (slowly in order to avoid a possible release of histamine that is associated to rapid IV administration), IM, SC, intraarticularly, epidurally or by continuous infusion. It provides analgesia for 2 to 4 hours in dogs and 6 to 8 hours in cats.
- **Hydromorphone:** it has replaced oxymorphone due to its lower price. It produces more sedation than oxymorphone but its effects last shorter. It produces excellent analgesia when combined with acepromazine. It does not cause histamine release.
- **Oxymorphone:** it is usually administered in combination with butorphanol. No hyperthermy has been observed after its administration in cats. As opposed to morphine, it does not release histamine liberation. It can be administered IV, IM or SC.

The two drugs that are described next are considered less powerful than the opioid agonist drugs previously mentioned. They are partial agonist (buprenorphine) or opioid agonist-antagonist drugs (butorphanol):

- **Butorphanol:** effective mainly in visceral pain treatment, derived from a cystitis or enteritis for example. It does not give very good results in somatic pain treatment. It provides analgesia for 30 minutes to 2.5 hours in cats and dogs. It seems to be more useful as a sedative (in particular when combined with acepromazine) and antitussive than as an analgesic.
- **Buprenophine:** the alkaline pH (8 and 9) of a cat's mouth makes the absorption of this drug easier, which is why it is very effective in this species compared to other species whose mouth's pH is neutral. It provides more analgesia in cats than morphine and oxymorphone. One of its disadvantages is that it takes approximately 30 minutes to take effect. In humans, it is possible to use buprenorphine transdermal patches to treat patients with cancer. It provides an analgesia of 4 to 8 hours in dogs and cats.

If the administration of an opioid drug is not enough to eliminate pain, it can be combined with other analgesic drugs such as NSAIDs, a continuous infusion of lidocaine, ketamine, an α_2-agonist or with a fentanyl patch. Combining these drugs will allow a reduction in the dosis of opioid required by reducing the appearance of dysphoric behaviours.

NSAIDs

General considerations

They inhibit the production of inflammation mediators (prostaglandins and thromboxanes) from arachidonic acid, responsible for the nociceptors' sensitivity in damaged tissue, by inhibiting the activity of the cyclooxygenase. When a cell is damaged it releases arachidonic acid. This substance is turned into different inflammation mediators by the action of the cyclooxygenase. There are two types of cyclooxygenase, COX-1 and COX-2. COX-1 is responsible for producing prostaglandins that will support some functions of the organism (maintaining gastric mucosal integrity, platelet function and kidney autoregulation), while COX-2 is associated to the production of prostaglandins related to inflammation.

NSAIDs act at peripheral and central level. At central level, they inhibit the transmission of pain within the spinal cord and, at peripheral level, they reduce pain associated to inflammation.

The development of COX-2-specific drugs has reduced adverse effects significantly, although it has recently been observed that COX-2 is involved in other processes (table 15).

Two disadvantages have to be taken into account. Firstly, their therapeutic margins are lower when compared to opioids and α_2-antagonists. Secondly, there are no antagonist drugs available to reverse their effects. However, in comparison with opioids, they provide a longer analgesia.

Table 15. Types of NSAIDs according to their specifity for COX-1 and COX-2.

TYPES OF NSAIDS	ACTION	DRUGS
Non specific	Inhibit COX-1 as much as or more than COX-2.	Aspirin. Phenylbutazone. Flunixin. Ibuprofen. Ketoprofen.
COX-2-specific	Inhibit COX-2 more than COX-1.	Carprofen. Meloxicam.
Coxibs (COX-2-specific)	High specificity for COX-2.	Robenacoxib. Rofecoxib. Firocoxib. Mavacoxib.
Dual inhibitors	Inhibit both COX-1 and COX-2.	Tolfenamic acid.

Most common side effects

The side effects are due to the inhibition of COX-1. They produce a higher toxicity in the feline species because of its lower capacity to glucoronidate these drugs. The effects they produce are:

- Ulcers, gastrointestinal haemorrhages, diarrhoea. These side effects can be prevented by administering a synthetic prostaglandin (e.g. misoprostol).
- Reduction of platelet aggregation.
- Kidney disorders (mainly in cats): interstitial nephritis, acute renal failure.
- Increased blood pressure.
- Liver failure (paracetamol).

Most used NSAIDs

- **Meloxicam:** COX-2-specific NSAID, enolic derivative. Used mainly in the treatment of musculoskeletal pain. Considered one of the safest NSAIDs. Provides analgesia for 24 hours. Its palatability is high even for cats. It can be administered orally or by injection.
- **Carprofen:** this drug is considered a weak inhibitor of the COXs. It is administered once a day and provides for 24 hours in dogs and 48 hours in cats.
- **Ketoprofen:** powerful anti-inflammatory and analgesic used to treat short-lasting pain in cats and dogs. As it is a powerful inhibitor of COX-1, it can interfere with platelet function.
- **Robenacoxib:** also used to treat musculoskeletal pain in cats.
- **Mavacoxib:** it is a coxib-class NSAID that acts on COX-2. It is used for the long-term treatment of pain and inflammation associated with a degenerative articular disease.

α_2-agonists

General considerations

These drugs act on α_2-adrenoceptors associated to the sympathetic nervous system. They produce analgesia, sedation, muscular relaxation and have an anxiolytic effect. They are metabolised in the liver and are eliminated by the kidney.

Atipamezol can be used in order to reverse their effects. If it is administered intravenously, this should be done slowly (2-3 minutes) since a rapid administration of atipemazol can induce hypotension. It is preferable to use the intramuscular route. They should not be used with atropin or other muscarinic drugs.

Side effects

- Cardiovascular: peripheral vasoconstriction, physiological bradychardia, hypertension (during the first 7-8 minutes).
- Decreased respiratory rate.
- Vomiting.
- Decreased intestinal motility.
- Moderate increase in blood glucose level.
- Moderate increase in urine production.

Most used α_2-agonists

- **Medetomidine:** pure agonist. It can be combined with butorphanol both in dogs and cats and with ketamin in cats. Its action lasts for about 60-90 minutes. It can be used in continuous infusion. Temperature should be monitored since this drug can occasionally cause hypothermy. It should not be administered in patients with a cardiovascular disease, craneal trauma or with hypovolemia.
- **Xylazine:** partial agonist. Less specific than medetomidine. Provides analgesia for 1 to 4 hours.

Local anaesthetics

General considerations

They act by blocking pain transmission in the nociceptive fibres, therefore providing analgesia in the area where they have been injected. These drugs block sodium channels, preventing the transmission of the pain stimulus to the central nervous system. They can be administered in different forms, topically or injected in a specific area (e.g. epidural analgesia, infiltration into the bone fracture area, etc.) (table 16). In addition, they can be used to block the nerves of a specific region (e.g. at the intercostal level). Nowadays, it is common to use epidural anaesthesia combining drugs such as lidocaine or bupivacaine with morphine. Another option is to inject the local anaesthetics into the wound or simply bathe the wound with them.

Lidocaine can be administered in continuous infusion in dogs, which will allow a reduction of the amount of anaesthetic used. This practice should be avoided in cats because of a possible cardiovascular depression.

Research focuses on the use of lidocaine transdermal patches in cats. In a study conducted in 2008, it was observed that transdermal patches could be useful to relieve the pain derived from minor skin injuries.

2

Table 16. Application routes for local analgesic agents.

Topical	• The application of a 10% lidocaine spray provides analgesia of the mucosa with a maximum depth of 2 mm for 15-20 minutes, 1-2 minutes after applying. • Use of cream for the skin (lidocaine + procaine) that provides analgesia for 1 hour.
Local infiltration	• Subcutaneous administration of small amounts of the local anaesthetic. Very useful, for example, to suture small wounds or carry out biopsies.
Local infiltration to block an area	• Can be useful to block all the nerves in the area when injected at the base of a limb.
Intravenous regional anaesthesia	• To obtain an analgesia (of a duration of less than 2 hours) of the distal part of the limbs.
Specific nerve block	• Used to block the infraorbital and mandibular nerve before dental surgeries.
Infiltration into a cavity	• The analgesic is injected into a cavity, for example, in the thoracic cavity, to reduce the pain derived from a thoracotomy.
Intraarticular analgesia	• Administration of the local analgesic into the joint.
Epidural administration	• Can be used as a complement to general anaesthesia to improve analgesia of hindquarter surgery. The drug is administered between the dura mater and the periosteum of the vertebra.

Side effects

- They are usually observed if the dosis is too high or if it has been adminstered intravenously. The most common side effects are convulsions and muscular spams.
- It is preferable not to use epidural anaesthesia (with a local anaesthetic, α_2-agonist or opioid) when there is a coagulopathy or sepsis.

Most used local anaesthetics

The most used local anaesthetics are **lidocaine** and **bupivacaine.** The effect of lidocaine appears before that of bupivacaine but its duration is shorter (2-3 hours against 4-5 hours) Diluting the drug in saline is recommended in order to obtain an appropriate volume. Both local anaesthetics can be combined to achieve a faster and longer-lasting effect.

Antagonists of NMDA receptor (N-methyl-D-aspartate)

General considerations

These drugs block the NMDA receptor, involved in the central sensitisation process. In human medicine, these drugs are used to treat neuropathic pain.

Most used drugs

- **Ketamine:** much used in cats as a sedative although there are few studies assessing its analgesic action. An interesting aspect is that this drug can only block the NMDA receptors if these have been opened by a previous noxious stimulus. This would explain why the effect observed is much lesser in healthy cats.
- **Amantadine:** this drug seems to be effective on chronic non-adaptive pain in dogs and cats. Together with an NSAID it seems to be effective to treat osteoarthritis in the canine species. There are no studies available for the feline species.

Psychoactive drugs

General considerations

Psychoactive substances act by modifying the levels of catecholamines and serotonin, two neurotransmitters involved in the transmission and modulation of pain. They can be of use when dealing with non-adaptive pain and traditional analgesics are not effective.

Most used psychoactive drugs

- **Selective serotonin reuptake inhibitor (fluoxetine):** they inhibit serotonin reuptake, thus increasing the levels of this neurotransmitter.
- **Tricyclic antidepressants (amitryptiline, clomipramine):** they inhibit serotonin and noradrenaline reuptake, thus increasing the levels of these neurotransmitters.
- **Monoamine oxydase inhibitors (selegiline):** they block monoamine oxydase thus increasing serotonin and noradrenaline levels.

The joint administration of drugs that increase serotonin levels can cause a serotonin syndrome (restlessness, hallucinations, irritability) as a result of an excess of serotonin. This can be prevented, for example, by avoiding the combined use of tramadol with a tricyclic antidepressant, a selective serotonin reuptake inhibitor or a monoamine oxidase inhibitor.

In addition to the psychoactive drugs previously mentioned, there is another group of drugs, benzodiazepines, which can be used occasionally when the patient shows fear and/or anxiety. These problems are known to be able to increase the pain suffered by the animal. Benzodiazepines, especially diazepam, can be uneffective in healthy dogs and cats if they are excited, although they are a good option in geriatric or weak animals.

Anticonvulsants

Some anticonvulsants also provide a certain degree of analgesia. In fact, they are occasionally used in human medicine to treat neuropathic pain.

Gabapentin is the most used anti-seizure drug to treat chronic pain. Its mechanism of action is still unclear, but it seems that it could inhibit the release of excitatory neurotransmitters, block calcium channels or activate the descending pathway that modulates pain. There are no specific studies available about its effectiveness in pain relief in either cats or dogs. However, some authors (Siao et al., 2009, Long term pain in cats) observed that this drug was effective to treat neuropathic pain in the canine species. The most common side effects are related to a depression of the central nervous system (vertigo, ataxia, drowsiness, etc.).

Mixed analgesics

Tramadol stands out in this group. This drug binds to the mu opioid receptors although it is not classified as an opioid drug. In addition, it inhibits serotonin and noradrenaline uptake, stimulates the endogenous inhibitory pathway and provides a slight anxiolytic effect. It is used in both human and veterinary medicine to treat chronic pain. It can be administered orally or intravenously. The main problem for its oral administration in the feline species is its bitter taste.

> The oral administration of drugs in the cat is very complicated and, in most species, translates into a reduction of the drug plasmatic levels due to the hepatic metabolism. There is an exception however, tramadol. This drug has some analgesic effect with a good oral biodisponibility.

The combination of analgesics if the most effective way of obtaining a good and longer-lasting analgesia. Some examples of combinations can be seen in Appendix 1 and the doses of the drugs most commonly used in Appendix 2.

Handling and housing conditions

It is important to handle the animal gently to reduce stress and prevent any problems of fear, anxiety or aggressiveness. These problems can increase pain and this pain can in turn increase these negative emotional states.

In those cases when the animal must be hospitalised, it is important to minimise manipulations as well as diagnostic tests. Sedating the animal can make the placement of a catheter and the carrying out of tests easier by preventing the animal from getting more stressed.

It is important to take the needs of each species into account in the hospitalisation area. We need to bear in mind that staying at the hospital means a high level of stress, especially for cats. Fearful behaviours, aggressiveness or anorexia can appear as a consequence of being handled, pain or simply as a result of the "stressful stay".

The placement of a bandage can occasionally be very uncomfortable for the cat and the licking of the area is a sign of discomfort rather than pain. If we take into account that it was observed in a study that the placement of a bandage caused an increase in urinary cortisol, we could think that this is a stressful measure for cats.

We must remember that food neophobia, that is to say, the rejection of new food, is a behaviour that is much more marked in the cat than in the dog. Neophobia is usually much more significant when the cat is in an unknown environment (e.g: hospital).

The following considerations can be taken into account:

- The cat and dog hospitalisation areas should be separated. If this is not possible, avoid at least visual contact (fig. 1).
- The use of pheromone diffusers (synthetic feline facial pheromone and dog-appeasing pheromone) to reduce stress and improve recovery.
- In the cages for cats:
    - If the state of the animal allows it, place a litter tray with very low borders (to make the access easier, especially in geriatric or weak animals).
    - Offer a place where the animals can hide (figs. 2 and 3).
    - If the size of the cage allows it, place a platform since tridimensional space is very important to cats.
- In the cages for dogs:
    - Place an object that is familiar to the dog (its basket, blanket, etc.).

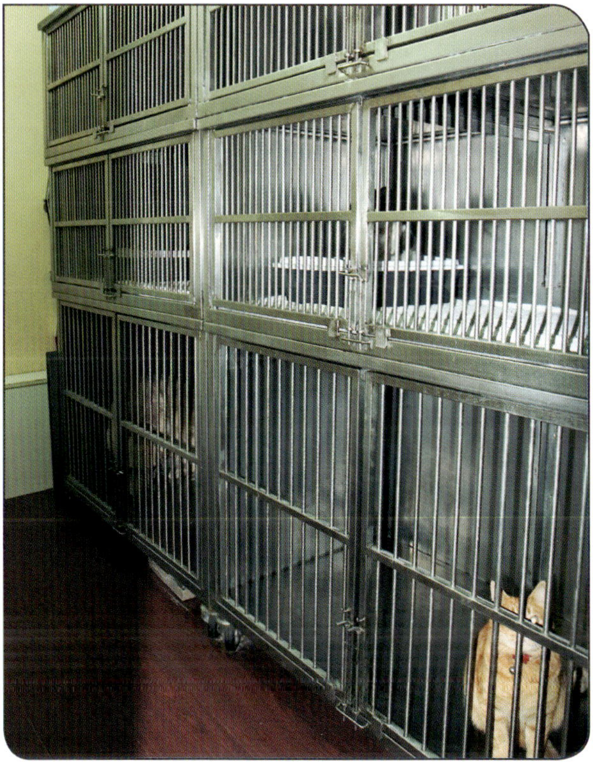

Figure 1. Hospital area. The location of the cages prevents visual contact between cats and dogs.

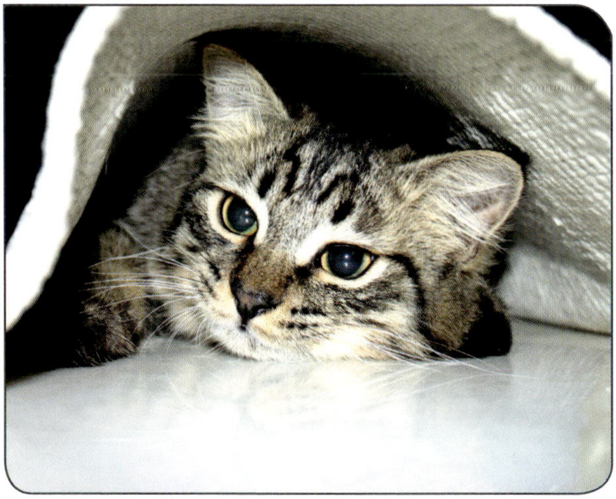

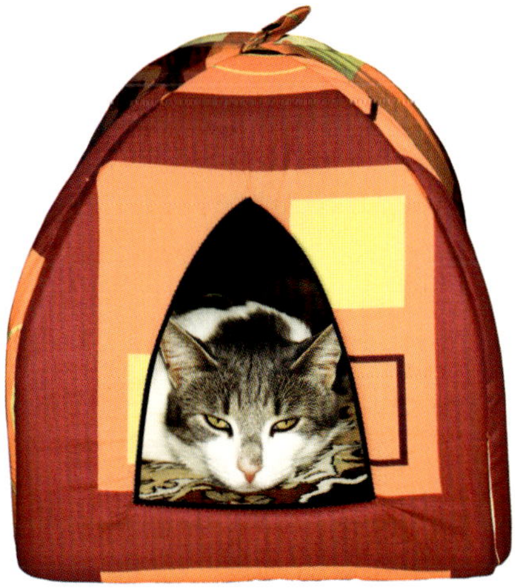

Figures 2 and 3. Cats will be much more calm if they have a place where they can hide during hospitalisation.

Nutraceuticals

No scientific studies confirming their usefulness to reduce articular inflammation and help in cartilage repair have been published in the veterinary field. However, in human medicine, a study comparing a group of patients suffering from knee arthritis who took glucosamine sulfate for 3 years with a group of people with the same ailment who took a placebo for the same period of time was recently published. It was observed that the group who had taken the neutraceutical had a significant improvement of their clinical signs, including pain.

Some nutraceuticals are used to treat feline intersitial cystitis. This problem is the result of the combination of physical and stress factors. The most common symptom in cats that suffer from this problem is unappropriate elimination. These animals excrete lower amounts of glycosaminoglycans. These changes in the bladder wall allow urine to be in contact with the nerve endings that supply the bladder, thus causing the release of neurotransmitters and local neurogenic inflammation, with the consequent pain. It seems that the administration of glycosaminoglycans could be effective as a complement to other handling, diet and pharmaceutical measures that the treatment includes.

Other therapies

Holistic therapies have recently become very popular. The main problem in the use of these therapies is the lack of scientific studies available. Acupuncture is the only therapy included in this group for which studies have been carried out. Placing needles in specific points could reduce muscle spams and induce the release of certain neurotransmitters.

APPENDIX

Appendix 1

Analgesic protocols.

PREDICTED LEVEL OF PAIN	PREOPERATIVE ANALGESIA	POSTOPERATIVE ANALGESIA
Mild	Pure/partial agonist opiod or NSAID.	Pure/partial agonist opioid or NSAID.
Mild to moderate	Agonist opioid + NSAID +/- α_2-agonist +/- epidural analgesia o local anaesthetic infiltration.	If necessary, one or more of these drugs: • Pure/partial agonist opioid. • NSAID. • Microdoses of α_2-agonist in infusion.
Moderate to severe	Pure opioid agonist (consider dosis during surgery) + NSAID + epidural analgesia epidural with bupivacaine or morphine + local anaesthesia of the nerve or regional block +/- ketamine or microdoses of α_2-agonist in infusion during surgery.	Agonist opioid. In addition, if necessary: • Higher or more frequent doses of the opioid. • Epidural analgesia. • Local anaesthesia (e.g.: inside the cavity). • Ketamine or microdoses of α_2-agonist in infusion.

Appendix 2

Doses of most used drugs in the dog and cat.

DRUG	DOG (mg/kg)	CAT (mg/kg)	ROUTE OF ADMINISTRATION
Morphine	0.1	0.1-.3	IV, IM
Hydromorphone	–	0.05-0.1	IV, IM
Butorphanol	0.2-0.5	0.1-0.4	IV, IM
Buprenorphine	0.01-0.03	0.01-0.02	IV, IM
Fentanyl	0.01-0.02	0.005-0.01 25 µg/hour	IV Transdermal patch
Ketoprofen	2	1-2	SC
Meloxicam	0.2 followed by 0.1	0.3 followed by 0.1	SC, IV, PO
Carprofen	4	1-4	SC
Mavacoxib	2, repeat after 14 days and then every month	–	PO
Ketamine	–	2	IV
Lidocaine	2-4	2-4	Local anaesthesia
Bupivacaine (infiltration)	2	2	Local anaesthesia
Amitriptyline	1-2	–	PO
Amantadine	3-5	3-5	PO
Tramadol	2-5	1-2	PO

Bibliography

GRANT, D. Pain management in small animals. *A manual for Veterinary Nurses and Technicians*. Elsevier, 2006.

GREGORY, N.H. Relationships between pathology and pain severities: a review. *Animal Welfare*, 2010; vol. 19. HELLYER, P., RODAN, I., BRUNT, J., DOWNING, R., HAGEDORN, J.E., ROBERTSON, S.A. AAHA/AAFP Pain Management Guidelines for Dogs & Cats. *Journal of the American Animal Hospital Association*, 2007; vol. 43.

LAMONT, L.A. Multimodal pain management in veterinary medicine: the phisiologic basis of pharmacologic therapies. *Vet Med Small Anim*, 2008; vol. 38.

MATHEWS, K.A. Neuropathic pain in dogs and cats: if only they could tell us if they hurt. *Vet Med Small Anim*, 2008; vol. 38.

ROBERTSON, S.A. Assessment and management of acute pain in cats. *Journal of Veterinary and Critical Care*, 2005; vol. 15.

ROBERTSON, S.A., LASCELLES, D. Long-term pain in cats. How much do we know about this important welfare issue? *Journal of Feline Medicine and Surgery*, 2010; vol. 12.

ROBERTSON, S.A., TAYLOR, P.M. Pain management in cats-past, present and future. Part 2. Treatment of pain-clinical pharmacology. *Journal of Feline Medicine and Surgery*, 2004; vol. 6.

RODAN, I. Understanding feline behavior and application for appropriate handling and management. *Topics in Companion Animal Medicine*, 2010; vol. 25(4).

RODAN, I., SUNDAHL, E., CARNEY, H., GAGNON, A.C., HEATH, S., LANDSBERG, G., SEKSEL, K., YIN, S. AAFP and ISFM Feline-Friendly Handling Guidelines. *Journal of Feline Medicine and Surgery*, 2011; vol. 13.

SHAFFRAN, N. Pain Management: The veterinary technician's perspective. *Vet Clin Small Anim*, 2008; vol. 38.

STAFFORD, K. *The welfare of dogs*. Springer, The Netherlands, 2007.

TAYLOR, P.M., ROBERTSON, S.A. Pain management in cats-past, present and future. Part 1. The cat is unique. *Journal of Feline Medicine and Surgery*, 2004; vol. 6.

PAIN AND BEHAVIOURAL PROBLEMS

Aggressive behaviour and pain

Introduction

Aggressive behaviour is defined as a behaviour whose objective is to cause physical harm to another individual. It is a very complex behaviour which depends on several genetic and environmental factors. The role of pain, one of the most important physical factors in aggressive behaviour, will be analysed in this chapter.

Aggressive behaviour problems in dogs are very common, and, at least in reference centres, they are the main behavioural problem. For instance, according to the data collected by the APBC (*Association of Pet Behaviour Counsellors*), 56.4% of dogs have been treated for a problem of aggressive behaviour on at least one occasion.

Pain-related aggression problems represent approximately 2-3% of these problems. This figure is probably underestimated, since the fact that pain can cause aggressive behaviour is not always taken into account. Except the study conducted by Camps et al. (in press), there are no studies about the relationship between pain and aggressive behaviour in the canine species. A retrospective analysis of 12 cases of aggressive behaviour caused by pain was carried out in this study. Different elements were analysed, such as the cause of pain, whether there were antecedents of aggressive behaviour, the posture of the dog during the attack, the context in which the attack took place, as well as whether impulsivity was present or not. The normal aggression sequence usually includes a group of warning signs first (growling, teeth baring, hair bristling, etc.). The dog shows more or less subtle signs of aggressiveness that precede biting (fig. 1). In some cases, dogs can greatly reduce these signs or even eliminate them completely. In this case, we are faced with an impulsive attack. In the study, the cause of pain that was most frecuently identified was hip dysplasia. The dogs that were aggressive before suffering from the problem that caused their pain were more impulsive, reacted aggressively more often when they were handled and adopted a more defensive posture than the dogs that had never reacted aggressively before.

Figure 1. Normal aggresion sequence and aggression sequence in an impulsive dog.

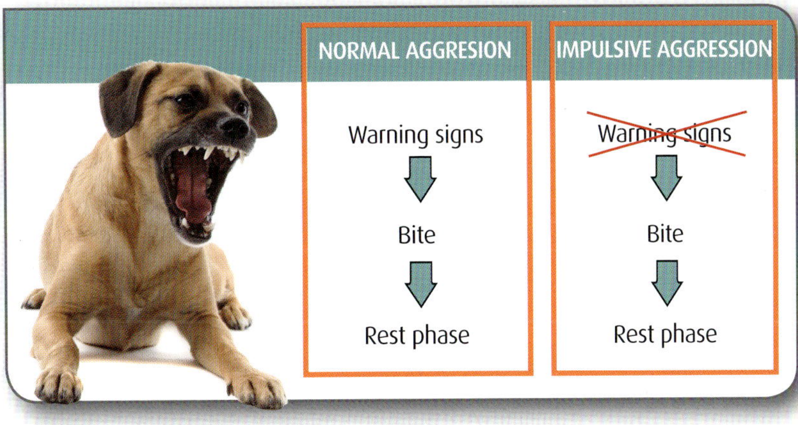

Specialists have developed differents classifications to categorise the different types of aggressive behaviour by basing themselves on the target of the attack, the context in which the aggression takes place and the position adopted by the animal during the aggressive episode. The current problem is the lack of consensus among specialists. The main point of disagreement is the terminology used to classify the different types of aggressive behaviour. For example, pain-related aggressive behaviour problems are included by some authors in the category of aggressive behaviour due to an organic cause. However, other specialists prefer using a separate category for these cases.

Although clinical classifications are more practical, the biological classification is the most objective one. This categorisation is based on the presence or absence of sympathetic activation. According to this criterion, aggressive behaviour can be divided in two types, affective and non-affective:

- In **affective-type aggressive behaviour** (which includes aggressive behaviour as a consequence of pain), there is a marked autonomous activation and the participation of structures such as the frontal cortex or the amygdala.
- In **non-affective-type aggressive behaviour** (also called non-emotional or predatory), there is no sympathetic activation. This aggressive behaviour is triggered by the movement of the prey and attacks are usually silent. The electric stimulation of the lateral hypothalamus triggers this type of aggressive behaviour.

Affective aggressive behaviour is in turn divided into **offensive aggressive behaviour** -whose objective is to obtain and/or protect a resource- and **defensive aggressive behaviour** -whose objective is to escape from a stimulus interpreted as a threat-. In the case of affective aggressive behaviour, animals adopt typical postures (fig. 2) and also often produce characteristic sounds.

In offensive aggressive behaviour, the animal stands tall and erect, its legs are extended, its ears are erect and forward, its tail is up and it stares and pulls its lips back showing only its incisors and canines. In defensive aggressive behaviour, its body is crouched, with its ears back and tail down, its back hair is raised and it pulls back its lips showing its molars too.

Figure 2. Offensive (a) and defensive (b) postures of the dog.

(a)

(b)

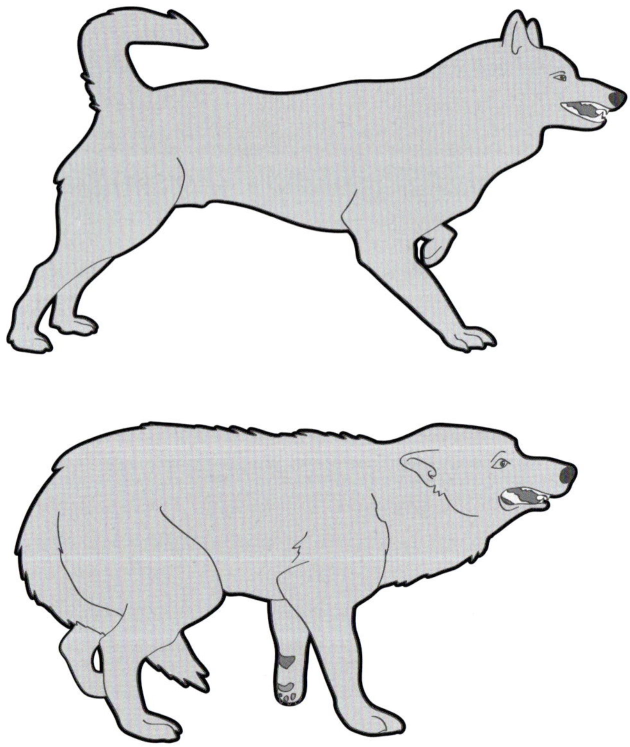

Mechanisms involved in the appearance of aggressive behaviour

It is widely documented that pain can cause aggressive behaviour. This aggressiveness can be triggered through three mechanisms.

Avoidance behaviour

Firstly, it may be a case of avoidance behaviour. In these cases, the animal reacts aggressively in order to avoid a particular handling procedure which had previously been painful. For example, a dog can bite when we try to lie it down if it is in pain due to a hip dysplasia problem.

Many authors claim that this avoidance reaction only occurs when the animal cannot escape from the aversive stimulus. However, some studies show that the application of a painful stimulus seems to increase the tendency to be aggressive towards a target, even when it is possible to escape from the aversive stimulus. For example, in a study carried out on people, in which they had to keep their hand submerged in very cold water, it was observed that the individuals who could decide when to remove their hands from the water were more hostile with their partner than those who could not do it (escape from the aversive stimulus).

It has also been demonstrated in other species that the application of an electric shock triggers an aggressive attack that is redirected towards another individual or an inanimate object. On some occasions, there seems to be an association between the aversive situation and the presence of another animal: the animal that receives the stimulus associates pain with the other individual and thus attacks it. On other occasions, it seems to be a reflex reaction that does not depend on a previous experience.

3

Stress

Secondly, stress plays an essential role in aggressive behaviour. The stimulation of the hypothalamic areas responsible for aggressive behaviour activates a stress response and the activation of the hypothalamus-pituitary-adrenal axis increases the tendency of an individual to be aggressive. It has been observed that acute stress induces analgesia while the effects of chronic stress on nociception are less predictable.

Some studies describe the appearance of analgesia after prolonged stress. However, hyperalgesia was observed after chronic stress in other works. It has been proposed that the opioidergic systems are activated when the stressful factor is weak or short-lasting, while non-opioid-related mechanisms are activated when the stressful stimulus is more powerful or lasts longer. But stress can also produce hyperalgesia depending on the type of stimulus. A reduction in pain sensitivity was observed in injured athletes or soldiers, whereas an increase in pain sensitivity was observed in people with neurasthenia and patients with fibromyalgia. An abnormal activity of the monoaminergic system seems to contribute to hyperalgesia, together with the P substance, neurokinin receptors, the calcitonin gene-related peptide, vasopressin and NMDA and AMPA receptors.

Some data confirms that the nociceptive effect of corticosteroids in chronic pain. Chronic corticosteroid treatments alter the expression of the neuropeptids involved in the transmission of the nociceptive stimulus at the spinal cord level, thus confirming the important role of glucocorticoid receptors in pain modulation at central level.

It should also be added that chronic stress is associated with a reduction in the serotonergic activity, which translates intro a greater tendency to show aggressiveness. Serotonin (5-HT, 5-hydroxytryptamine) is the neurotransmitter most involved in aggressive behaviour. This monoamine is synthesised from tryptophan, which is an essential amino acid. Serotonergic neurons are widely spread throughout the central nervous system.

There are at least three proofs that demonstrate the relationship between serotonin and aggressive behaviour:

1. Firstly, several studies have shown a negative correlation between the serotonin activity in the central nervous system and aggressive behaviour.
2. Secondly, the administration of drugs that increase the serotinin activity reduces aggressiveness.
3. Finally, the administration of a diet low in tryptophan which, as said before, is the precursor amino acid of serotonin, increases aggressive behaviour. A reduction in serotonergic activity in patients with chronic pain would therefore explain a greater tendency to react aggressively.

Reduction in physical activity

Thirdly, a reduction in activity can, although indirectly, trigger aggressive behaviour. It has been observed that a reduction in the physical activity of production animals and laboratory rodents is correlated with an increase in aggressive behaviour due to a reduction in serotonergic activity. The effect of exercise on the synthesis of this neurotransmitter is well-known. In fact, increasing physical activity is one of the recommendations that are occasionally given for dogs with aggressive behaviour problems, since an increase in the synthesis of serotonin after doing physical exercise has been demonstrated in many species.

3

SUMMARY

Aggressive behaviour can appear as a consequence of a learning process (avoidance behaviour) or due to a decrease in serotonin levels associated to chronic pain and/or reduced physical activity.

It should be remembered that serotonin is one of the neurotransmitters involved in the modulation of the nociceptive stimulus. At peripheral level, when there is tissue damage, serotonin is released from the platelets, mastocytes and endothelial cells endogenously. It has been observed that the exogenous administration of serotonin increases excitability of both Aδ and C fibres. In fact, the intradermal administration of low concentration 5-HT in the masseter muscle causes burning, pain and hyperalgesia. This suggests that in cases of tissue damage, serotonin would contribute to peripheral sensitisation. The 5-HT_{2A}, 5-HT_3 and 5-HT_7 peripheral receptors seem to be involved.

At central level, both electrical and chemical stimulation of the PAG (periaqueductal grey matter), located in the cerebral aqueduct and considered as the "centre of analgesia", induces the release of serotonin and consequently causes pain. The administration of serotonin in the spinal canal causes anti-nociception after the application of an acute noxious stimulus, while the administration of a serotonin antagonist reduces the analgesia induced by the stimulation of the nucleus raphe magnus, from where the serotonergic pathways that descend to the spinal cord are originated.

However, although its role is mainly inhibitory at central level, recent studies suggest that the descending serotonergic pathways could either play an inhibitory role or stimulate nociception depending on the type of nociceptive stimulus. The descending serotonergic pathways seem to have an inhibitory effect in cases of inflammatory pain, but they also seem to have a stimulating effect and contribute to central sensitisation in cases of tissue damage. This inhibitory or stimulating effect of serotonin could also depend on the type of serotonin receptor involved.

In fact, it was recently observed that the agonists of the 5-HT_{1A} and 5-HT_7 receptors or the agonists of the 5-HT_{2A} and 5-HT_3 receptors could be excellent candidates for the treatment of pain. In addition, some studies have shown that the individuals with a greater number of 5-HT_{1A} receptors express less pain.

SUMMARY
Most studies agree on the fact that acute stress induces analgesia and, although the results are more variable, that chronic stress is associated with hyperalgesia.

Treatment of pain-related aggressive behaviour problems

Use of drugs with analgesic properties

In chapter 2, we listed the drugs most commonly used to treat pain: opioids, NSAIDs, α_2-agonists, local anaesthetics, NMDA receptor antagonists and psychoactive drugs. As regards the latter ones, it should be highlighted that they are usually used to treat chronic pain. In fact, tricyclic antidepressants (TCAs) are the drugs of choice to treat neuropathic pain.

There are three main mechanisms through which TCAs provide analgesia:
- Firstly, by blocking sodium channels.
- Secondly, by blocking calcium ion channels.
- Thirdly, by blocking the reuptake of monoaminergic, serotonergic and noradrenergic neurotransmitters at central level, by increasing their availability.

We should remember that painful stimuli open ion channels, thus causing the nervous stimulus.

In addition to these three mechanisms, these drugs also have an analgesic effect as a result of their antihistamine action, their interaction with the opioid system and their action as antagonists of the N-methyl-D-aspartate receptor (one of the receptors to which glutamate, the main excitatory transmitter, binds).

3

Behaviour modification techniques

In the cases where there has been a negative association between, for example, a person and a specific painful manipulation, it may be necessary, in addition to using analgesics, to break this association by using behaviour modification techniques. By means of desensitisation and counter-conditioning technique, we can get a dog used to being approached and handled (see example).

EXAMPLE OF BEHAVIOUR MODIFICATION TECHNIQUE

Aggressive episode: a dog recovering from a hip surgery reacted aggressively when the owner tried to brush its lumbar area.

Technique: in this case, we will start the exercise by getting the dog used to the sight of the aversive stimulus (brush + owner) while distracting it with some food. If its attitude is good, we will give it the reward. The exercise will then be made more difficult by increasing the intensity of the aversive stimulus. If the dog does not react when the owner takes the brush, the next step is to get closer with the brush and stroke the animal with our hand, but without using the brush yet. We will later run the flat side of the brush (not the bristle or pin side) along its body and finally we will brush the dog.

It is very important to remember that it is necessary to create a pleasant and motivational atmosphere and reward the animal everytime its behaviour is positive. If at some point the dog shows signs of aggressive behaviour, we must not punish it but come back to the previous step instead.

Conclusions

The diseases most frequently associated with pain were listed in the previous chapter. It is important to apply an appropriate analgesic protocol to ensure pain control and thus avoid the appearance of aggressive behaviour. Furthermore, during a behavioural consultation, the diagnostic protocol must include a medical check-up that will allow us to rule out possible diseases the animal could suffer from and which may influence or be the direct cause of the aggressive behaviour showed by the animal.

Compulsive behaviour and pain

Introduction

On occasions, dogs and cats show repetitive behaviours which are known as compulsive behaviours and, as will be seen later, can be caused by pain. Some authors use the expression of obsessive-compulsive disorder because of its similarity to the disorder described in human medicine, in which the affected individuals repeatedly perform a behaviour in order to try to solve an obsessive thought (obsession). However, it is not known whether animals are able to have obsessions, so in this chapter we will refer to this disorder as compulsive behaviour.

How compulsive behaviour is developed

When a stressful, frustrating or conflict situation occurs, the animal can respond by performing a displacement behaviour, that is to say, a behaviour that does not make sense in this particular context. If the situation is not solved and becomes chronic, these displacement activities that appear sporadically can become repetitive and then compulsive or stereotyped. For example, a dog that cannot attack another dog walking past the house (due to the physical barrier of the fence) may feel frustrated and perform a displacement behaviour (for instance, chasing its tail). As the situation occurs every day, this behaviour is more and more frequent until it becomes compulsive and appears even if the triggering stimulus (the other dog) is no longer there.

Some studies suggest that genetically predisposed animals can develop stereotypies as a response to a stressful situation or an inappropiate environment. The fact that an animal may develop a compulsive disorder therefore depends on its genetic predisposition and the environment it is in.

Predisposing factors

Environmental factors

An inappropriate environment (box 1) can predispose the animal to develop such disorders.

Box 1. Examples of environmental factors which can contribute to the appearance of compulsive behaviours.

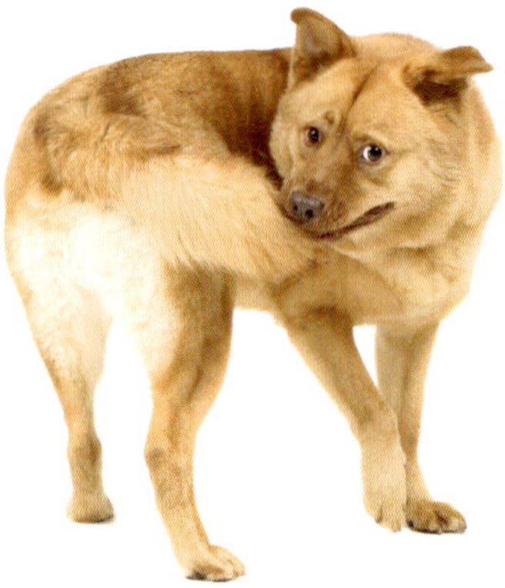

- **Lack of social contact:** no or little contact with owners or other dogs.
- **Lack of stimulation:** playing little with the dog, not walking it, etc.
- **Situations that cause frustration to the dog** (when its expectations are not met).
- **Situations of conflict** (when it has two opposite motivations).

Physical stimuli

In some cases, an animal can start licking a lesion because it is painful and/or it has pruritus and then continue to lick other parts of its body.

Learning

Owners tend to reinforce these disorders involuntarily as they try to calm down or distract the animal. Although this may initially work, what they are doing is encourage this behaviour since the animal learns that by performing this behaviour it receives its owners' attention.

Temperament

Some authors suggest that these problems appear more often in "anxious animals". In fact, in a study carried out at the animal behaviour clinic of Purdue University (Indiana, United States), it was observed that dogs with these disorders presented problems of pain-related aggressive behaviour more often than dogs with other behavioural problems.

Age

On average, this problem starts a little before 2 years old (it is similar in people, at around adolescence). However, it can appear at any age.

Genotype

In most compulsive behaviours, we can observe a genetic predisposition (table 1).

Table 1. Breed predisposition to compulsive behaviours.

BREED	COMPULSIVE BEHAVIOUR
Doberman Pinscher	Flank licking.
English Bull Terrier	Walking in circles, placing their head under or between objects and freezing.
Staffordshire Bull Terrier	Walking in circles.
German Shepherd	Tail chasing.
Australian Shepherd	Tail chasing.
Miniature Schnauzer	Looking at their hind part.
Border Collie	Hallucinations, chasing shadows.
Giant breeds	Persistent licking.
Siamese and Burmese	Wool sucking.

Modified from the *Manual of canine and feline behavioural medicine*, BSAVA, 2010; pp. 237.

3

Relationship between pain and compulsive behaviour

Chronic pain is a source of stress. It has previously been mentioned that stress can trigger the appearance of a displacement behaviour, which can become compulsive if the situation does not improve.

In human medicine, several studies have been published in which chronic pain has been linked to the expression of anxiety. For example, some data obtained in 2003 in the United States indicates that the individuals who suffer from chronic pain show more anxiety disorders than the general population (35% against 17%). This category includes obsessive-compulsive disorders, post-traumatic stress, phobias or generalised anxiety. More specifically, in a study conducted in 1991 with 97 people who suffered from chronic back pain, 28.5% of them presented an anxiety problem and 8.2% showed an obsessive-compulsive disorder.

Diseases that can trigger a compulsive disorder associated with pain

Neurological

- It was observed that some animals suffering from lumbosacral stenosis or cauda equina syndrome walk in circles in a compulsive way (circling).
- Sensory neuropathies can induce compulsive paw chewing or licking. In this pathology, sensitivity to pain in the areas distal to the limb is reduced.
- The amputation of the tail can cause the development of neuromas which, as mentioned in the previous chapters, are associated with chronic pain. This pathology can trigger compulsive tail chasing.

Dermatological

Any dermatological lesion that causes pain and/or pruritus can trigger licking which may then become a compulsive behaviour (e.g.: acral lick dermatitis, fig. 3). In addition, these lesions can increase stress and thus the probability to develop this disorder.

Figure 3. Dog with acral lick dermatitis.

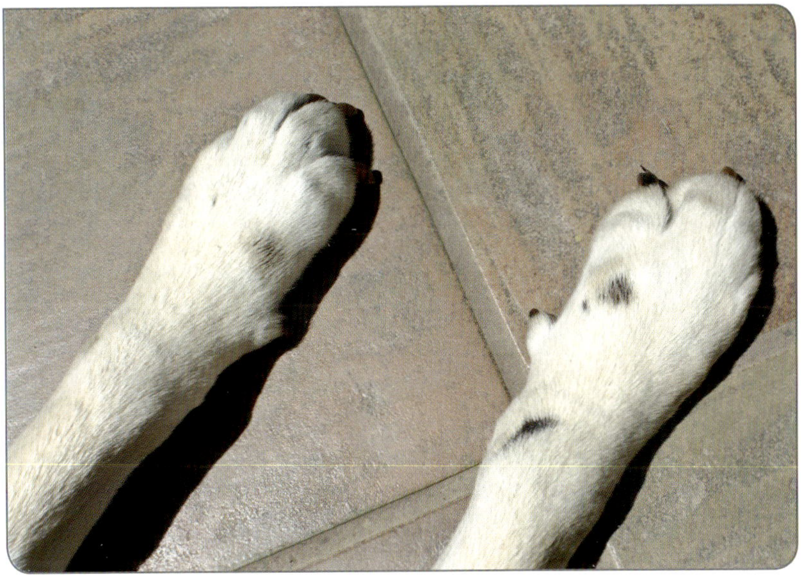

Musculoskeletal

Tail fractures or arthritis can make the animal pay more attention to the painful area and subsequently develop a compulsive behaviour.

Urinary system diseases

Feline interstitial cystitis is a disease of the lower urinary tract that is painful to the cat. It is the result of the combination of both physical factors and stress. In addition to a problem of inappropriate urination (the cat stops using its litter tray correctly), there are two compulsive behaviours that can be associated with this disease:

- **Psychogenic alopecia:** excessive grooming of the abdomen, inguinal and/or dorsolumbar areas.
- **Feline hyperesthesia syndrome:** excessive licking, vocalisations, increased activity, muscle spams, self-directed aggressive behaviour, etc.

Treatment

The key treatment points of compulsive behaviour are reflected in the following table.

TREATMENT OF COMPULSIVE BEHAVIOUR

1. **Eliminate or reduce stress as much as possible**
   It is very important to eliminate the source of stress (e.g.: solve a hierarchy conflict between two dogs) or reduce the exposure of the animal to it (e.g.: if seeing other cats in the garden is a cause of stress, we should prevent the animal from having access to that particular window).
2. **Environmental enrichment**
   This measure is indispensable in those cases where the lack of stimulation can have an influence on the development of the problem. Increasing the time spent on physical activity (walks, playing, etc.) and social contact are some options.
3. **Correcting the owners' management of their pet**
   Establishing a routine and a coherent management. It is very important to eliminate rewards and punishments that are not properly applied.
4. **Drug therapy**
   These disorders are very heterogeneous. Alterations of serotonergic, dopaminergic or glutamatergic transmission have been described. Furthermore, some studies describe high levels of β-endorphines in patients with these disorders.
   The use of pyschoactive drugs is common in chronic cases and will facilitate the application of the other measures. The treatment usually starts with a serotonergic drug (fluoxetine or clomipramine).

The patient may not respond to the medical treatment with serotonergic drugs. In these cases, several options are possible.

- Administering a narcotic antagonist such as naltrexone (only available in oral form) since there could be an internal reinforcement caused by endorphines. The problem is that few studies have been carried out in the canine species.
- Administering a dopaminergic antagonist such as haloperidol. However, the dosis for dogs has not been clearly determined and side effects are frequent and serious.
- Administering a NMDA receptor antagonist (memantine) that will act on glutamatergic neurotransmission. There seems to occasionally be a positive response to these drugs in people with these disorders. In a study conducted in dogs with a compulsive problem, it was observed that 64% of the cases responded positively to the administration of memantine (occasionally combined with fluoxetine) as well as to behaviour modification techniques. Nevertheless, more studies are necessary to obtain more conclusive results.

Pain and fear, phobia and anxiety

General concepts

It is important to differentiate the concepts of fear, phobia and anxiety. In human medicine, fear is defined as the apprehension caused by a stimulus, which can either be animated or not, or a specific situation. However, in veterinary medicine, the concept is more complex, and perhaps for this reason, it is defined in many different ways. Many of these definitions focus on the protective aspect of fear and do not exclude each other. Some examples would be: the state of alarm or terror, an unpleasant emotion caused by danger, the emotional state in which an animal is when it expects pain, the hypothetical state in which the brain and the neuroendocrine system are in a threat situation, etc. Fear is included in primary emotions, and one of the most objective definitions seems to be the one that describes fear as an emotional (psychophysiological) response which occurs as a response to a perceived danger (Jones B., 1997). In short, fear is a primary emotion which, whatever the definition may be, is unpleasant for the animal.

The response to fear is highly adaptive, and therefore, essential to survival. In this case, the intensity of the response is proportional to the stimulus. Fear is a normal and self-protective response which occurs in the presence of stimuli that are potentially dangerous for the animal. It can generally be expressed in three different ways: through freezing, fleeing or aggression, which are known as the three Fs (*freeze*, *flight* and *fight*) and which will be analysed in more detail later in this chapter.

In human psychiatry, a phobia is described as an "irrational" fear, since it is disproportionate to the actual threat. And although some authors prefer not to use this definition in veterinary medicine, as it is impossible to know whether what the animal is experiencing is a real threat or not, the truth is that a similar definition can be given. In short, a phobia is:

1. An intense fear response that is out of context and/or disproportionate to what would be expected in relation to the degree of threat.
2. A response that limits the animal's normal behaviour.
3. An "all or nothing" response: when a particular threshold is reached, the fear response is very intense and does not depend on the intensity of the threat.
4. The phobic response, as opposed to fear, remains after the stimulus that causes the threat has disappeared.

In short, in the case of a phobia, as opposed to fear, the response is not adaptive. The mechanism through which phobias are developed is not well-known; however, it is known that some animal seem prediposed to suffer from them. Furthermore, many expositions to the stimulus are often necessary to generate a phobic response in laboratory conditions; nonetheless, many dogs or cats can naturally develop phobias with only one exposition. Phobic behaviour which cannot be associated with aversive situations that have happened to the animal is even often observed.

Finally, anxiety is defined as the fear response that is generated when a threat is expected or in the presence of an objectively inexistent danger. As opposed to what happens with fear, in which the feeling of apprehension is intense and the recovery is fast when the threatening stimulus has disappeared, a non-specific state of apprehension characterised by a persistent sympathetic stimulation and hypervigilance is observed in the anxiety response. The anxious dog is tense and physiologically prepared for a possible threat that it is not able to predict. In addition, in many cases this threat is not real and never actually occurs. Occasionally, this state can become more and more frequent and be expressed in many different situations in the animal's daily life. This chronic state of anxiety can generate a state of chronic stress that will facilitate the appearance of other behavioural problems, including aggressive behaviours that are difficult to predict.

Factors involved in the appearance of fear

There are various factors that can facilitate the appearance of fear in an animal. The most important among them are:

1. The phylogenetic history of the species.
2. Individual genetic factors.
3. The socialisation period.
4. The experiences of the animal at the adult age.

Phylogenetic history of the species

On many occasions, adaptive fear appears due to stimuli that have a phylogenetic meaning for the species. Among them we can find pain, rapid changes of stimuli, loud noises, sudden movements, heights, water, fire and social or stimulating situations that are not familiar to the animal. It is therefore important to point out that pain itself is a phylogenetic source of fear for cats and dogs.

Individual genetic factors

Most of the behavioural genetic traits are probably difficult to define and quantify. In general, the estimated inheritability is low, and it can even be said that in many cases it is not significatively different from zero. The only known important exception so far is precisely the "fear character". This refers to the tendency of the animal to show a fear response when it is in a foreign environment. The estimations regarding the inheritability of this character in dogs often vary between 0.4-0.5, which means that the tendency of a dog to show fear depends approximately as much on genetics as on its environment. In other words, as opposed to what occurs with most behavioural characters, the animals that are descended from individuals with a fearful character will more easily develop fear behaviours.

Assistance dogs are a good example of the importance of the appearance of fear behaviours at the adult age and genetics. The main cause for rejecting an animal is the appearance of fear behaviours. This basically leads to two problems: animal welfare on the one hand, and financial costs on the other, since most dogs are rejected after completing the whole training process. With the aim of solving these problems, there are preliminary genetic studies that are designed to genetically identify the animals as regards their ability to serve as assistance dogs, depending on the fear character (Takeuchi Y., 2007).

Socialisation period

The third important factor to take into account is the socialisation period. The developmental periods of cats and dogs are divided into the neonatal period, the transitional period, the socialisation period and the juvenile period (fig. 4). The socialisation period lasts from the 3rd to the 12th week of life in the case of dogs and from the 2nd to the 7th week of life in the case of cats, although there can be variations depending on the breed and the individual. According to some authors, we can distinguish between primary and secondary socialisation, which would last from the 3rd to the 5th week and from the 5th to the 12th week respectively in dogs.

It is widely accepted that the socialisation period starts with the maturation of the vision and hearing senses, which are not functional from birth. Although there are several theories about which processes determine the end of this period, the most accepted one points out that the socialisation period ends with the maturation of the pathways that control the fear response. From the 8th week the animal starts to show a fear response, and from the 10th-12th weeks the response is so intense that the dog is reluctant to explore new stimuli.

A very fast development of the CNS, which allows rapid progress in behaviour, takes place during the socialisation period. The first social behaviours typical of the adult age appear, as well as an intense exploratory behaviour and play. In addition, the first dominant-submissive relationships establish themselves, detachment from the mother starts and abilities that are important at the adult age, such as body language and bite inhibition, are acquired.

However, one of the most important processes that takes place during socialisation is habituation to stimuli. Given its high exploratory behaviour and lack of fear, the puppy is in contact with a multitude of stimuli. The experience with these stimuli during this period will mark the puppy's attitude towards them from the age of three months. If an animal is isolated from any environmental

Figure 4. Developmental periods of dogs and cats.

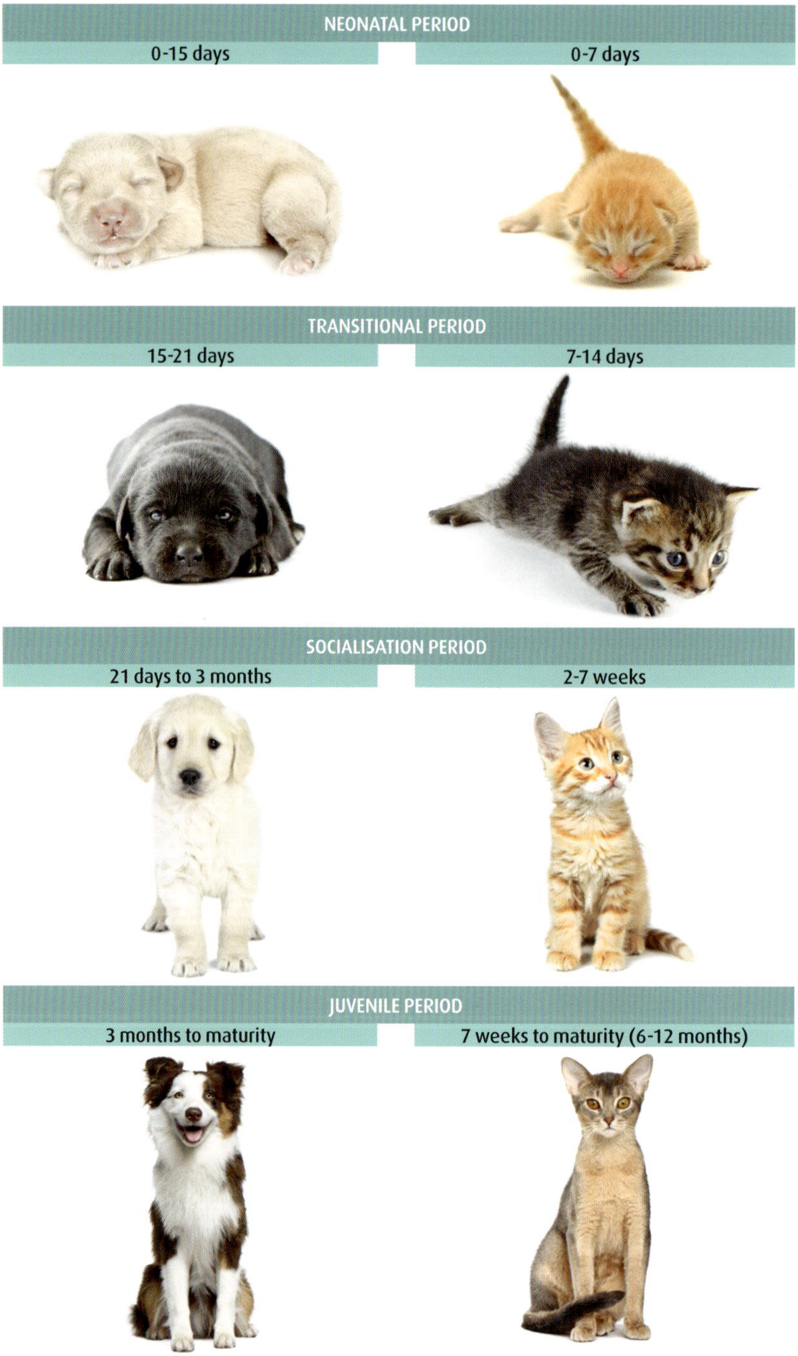
NEONATAL PERIOD
0-15 days
0-7 days
TRANSITIONAL PERIOD
15-21 days
7-14 days
SOCIALISATION PERIOD
21 days to 3 months
2-7 weeks
JUVENILE PERIOD
3 months to maturity
7 weeks to maturity (6-12 months)

stimulation during this period, this facilitates the development of serious behavioural problems, such as aggressiveness, repetitive behaviours, phobic fears, etc. On the other hand, if the animal is in contact with different stimuli during the socialisation period, it will not show any fear in their presence later, and will be cautious in the presence of other stimuli with which it has had no experience. Obviously, if the contact with these stimuli is negative during the socialisation period, it will also show fear in their presence as an adult.

Several studies compared the fear reaction of two groups of animals. Group 1 received a good stimulation during the socialisation period, while group 2 was not well socialised. When comparing the fear reaction (measurement of neophobia) that both groups showed as adults in the presence of a stimulus to which none of them had been habituated, group 1 (good socialisation) responded with less intensity than the group of poorly socialised animals (Krushinkii K.V., 1960).

However, some studies indicate that excessive stimulation during the socialisation period ("inundating the animal with stimuli") could be detrimental to the animal's development since it would facilitate the appearance of fear behaviours.

From a clinical point of view, this period is of particular importance since it is a period in which a positive contact with many different stimuli is necessary but, as a disadvantage, the animal's vaccination programme has not been completed yet. Therefore, in order to avoid any problems related to poor socialisation, it is possible to attend *puppy parties®* that help to facilitate the correct socialisation of puppies in a controlled manner and habituate them to common stimuli such as people, which is particularly important in the case of children and elderly people, car noises, fireworks or storms, etc.

The behavioural problems derived from poor socialisation can be treated when they are adults; however, although there can be improvements, the prognosis is guarded or poor.

Experiences of the animal at the adult age

The last important factor involved in the appearance of fear behaviours is the experience as an adult. Fear can be induced by a great variety of unconditional and conditional stimuli. * Animals are able to create associations between unconditional stimuli (US) that cause fear per se and other conditional stimuli (CS) which are often presented together with unconditional stimuli. In other words, and as an example, when dogs visit the vet, they are often suffering from a painful condition (US), and this painful experience is associated with some specific contextual elements (the white coat, a particular smell, the examination table, etc. -CS-).

When this happens repeatedly, and although there may be only one association, learning through classical conditioning takes place, which leads to the CS being able to produce the response in the absence of the US (in this case, pain). In these circumstances, the animal may therefore show fear only due to the presence of the CS (white coat, examination table, characteristic smell of the consultation room, etc.).

Finally, there is also a relationship between fear and operating conditioning which will be analysed further on. However, to summarise, there are numerous studies which show a high correlation between the use of positive punishment (a type of operating conditioning) and fear behaviours, and even aggression caused by fear and frustration.

*Traditionally, we talked about "conditioned" and "unconditioned" stimuli. However, this terminology is attributed to a bad translation from Russian to English that has remained through time. The correct terminology would be "condtional" and "unconditional". In fact, it is more intuitive, since it refers to the fact that the US by itself, with no condition, can induce the response (unconditional). However, for the CS to induce a response, it needs to have previously occurred together with the US on one or more occasions, that is to say, it needs a condition.

Neurophysiology of fear

The important structures of the CNS involved in the fear response are (fig. 5):

1. **Amygdala:** it is a subcortical region that plays a crucial role in processing the information from reinforcement and punishment in conditioned fear. The connections between the amygdala and the cortical structures (especially the orbitofrontal cortex) are important for the association of reinforcement and punishment (Cohen, 1980). In human medicine, functional neuroanatomical tests have demonstrated that in the presence of fear situations, the amygdala is activated and its electrical stimulation produces feelings of fear and apprehension. In addition, lesions in the amygdala eliminate the ability of someone to recognise the signs of fear.

   It has also been shown in animals that electrical stimulation of the amygdala produces a range of physiological and behavioural responses that indicate fear. Furthermore, a lesioned amygdala in animals results in the absence of fear, whose evaluation is based on the avoidance of danger situations.
2. **Hippocampus**: it analyses the novelty of the stimulus (important, for example, in neophobia), as well as the previous associations that the animal may have done with previous negative experiences and that particular stimulus. That is to say, it plays a crucial role in processing complex stimuli, since it helps to "bring together" the different elements of a stimulus, thus producing a representation of it that can be associated to a US.

   The role of the hippocampus changes with time. When an organism is exposed to a complex stimulus for the first time, the hippocampus seems to be necessary to process the relationships between the stimuli. However, with time, this information seems to be stored in another place, probably in the cortex. As a result, a lesion of the hippocampus has lesser consequences if it occurs during the last stages of learning. In other words, the hippocampus is the important centre of short-term memory.

3. Finally, the **structures in charge of generating the responses** of all this circuit are multiple. The most important of them are:
   a. **Periaqueductal grey matter** (PAG): related to the organisation of the defensive response. It is associated with analgesia processes and changes in activity. Different parts of the PAG induce different changes. The lateral nucleus is involved in the fight-or-flight response, while the basolateral nucleus is related to the freeze response.
   b. **Reticular formation** (of the brainstem). It is a mediator in the startle response.
   c. **Hypothalamus:** partially responsible for the hormonal stress response of fear. The activation of the sympathetic response is mediated directly by the amygdala through the dorsal nucleus of the vagus nerve, and indirectly through the hypothalamus. The hypothalamic-pituitary-adrenal axis is activated. The activation response of the sympathetic nervous system, which is partly responsible for the fight-or-flight response, includes, in addition, an inhibition of the parasympathetic nervous system.

The neurotransmitters involved are:

1. **Noradrenaline:** it is a mediator in the behaviour and physiological reactions associated with the emotional fear response. It is released mainly in the locus coeruleus, frontal cortex and hypothalamus. The increase in the transmission of noradrenaline is linked to greater levels of excitement, awareness, vigilance and control of facial expressions.
   The activation of the β-adrenergic system is associated with the activation of short-term memory. The site of action of catecholamines for this purpose is the amygdala.
2. **Serotonin:** its role is not very clear. It increases in cases of fear and other situations that generate stress.
3. **Dopamine:** it is mainly released in the frontal cortex and the amygdala. It it also released in the brainstem, where the activating reticular system, which contains great amounts of dopamine and noradrenaline, is located. It is directly connected to the amygdala.
4. **GABA:** it has an inhibitory action on fear. It seems that serotonin acts by boosting GABA in these situations.

All these neurophysiological circuits generate the behavioural response of fear, which will be analysed in more detail later in this chapter (symptoms of fear).

Figure 5. Important structures of the CNS involved in the fear response (adapted from Domjan, 2003).

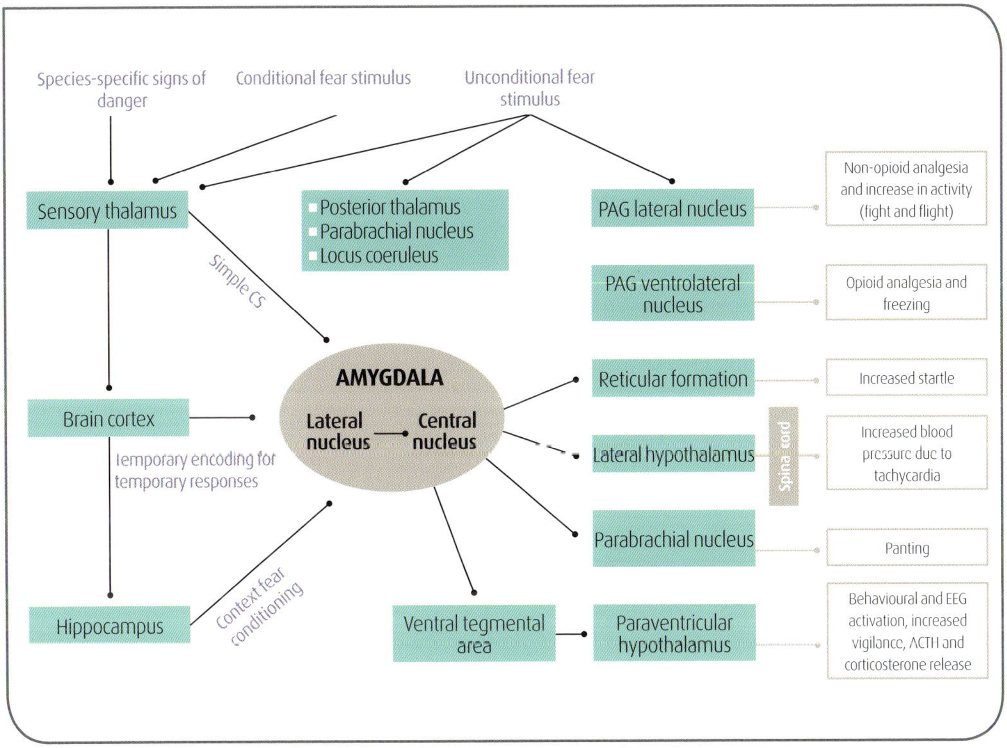

Mechanisms of fear induction caused by pain

There are two basic mechanisms through which pain can cause fear. First of all, pain acts as an unconditional stimulus which induces a fear response. In fact, the neurological pathways responsible for pain, fear and anxiety, are closely related anatomically as well as chemically and functionally. Therefore, when an animal is in a situation in which it experiences pain, it will try to create associations between the stimulus that causes pain and the neutral stimuli (CS) that may help it to predict a similar situation in the future. That is why when the conditioned contextual elements are present again later, the animal may show fear even in the absence of the initial US that caused pain. This learning process is very adaptive and allows the animal to avoid situations that can put its physical integrity at risk.

The second mechanism is not as intuitive and only seems to be demonstrated in the human species. It has been widely demonstrated that people who suffer from some painful condition, like animals, can generate an anxiety response. These people have a higher probability of showing a pessimistic perception of the environment (pessimistic cognitive bias), which makes initially neutral stimuli become potential (unreal) sources of pain and causes them to avoid initially innocuous stimuli (due to a reaction of fear at the prospect of them being able to cause pain) (Deghani et al., 2008).

Although there is no scientific evidence to back this up, this process could take place in a similar way in animals. Two clinical cases of dogs were presented (Lindley, 2012), in which a Labrador and a Boxer showed a problem of fear in the presence of rather unconventional stimuli and in addition, did not respond to the conventional treatment for a problem of fear. These animals were simultaneously diagnosed with chronic pain. Applying an analgesic treatment together with a treatment for fear solved the problems.

Finally, it should be highlighted that there are numerous studies in many different species, including dogs, that demonstrate that animals can show a more pessimistic or optimistic view of the environment. This is called positive or negative cognitive bias (optimistic or pessimistic, respectively). In fact, one of these studies showed that dogs suffering from separation anxiety (a behavioural condition in which the dog experiences an anxiety reaction when it cannot be with the owner), have a more pessimistic character than the average of the general population (Mendl et al., 2010). We could therefore expect other diseases, which are known to have the ability to cause an anxiety response like pain, to also cause a pessimistic perception of the environment. The generalised fear or anxiety response to other initially neutral stimuli described in human medicine may thus occur in animals too (fig. 6).

It is important to highlight that the use of learning techniques based on positive punishment induces fear in animals and should therefore always be avoided.

Figure 6. Environmental negative cognitive bias.

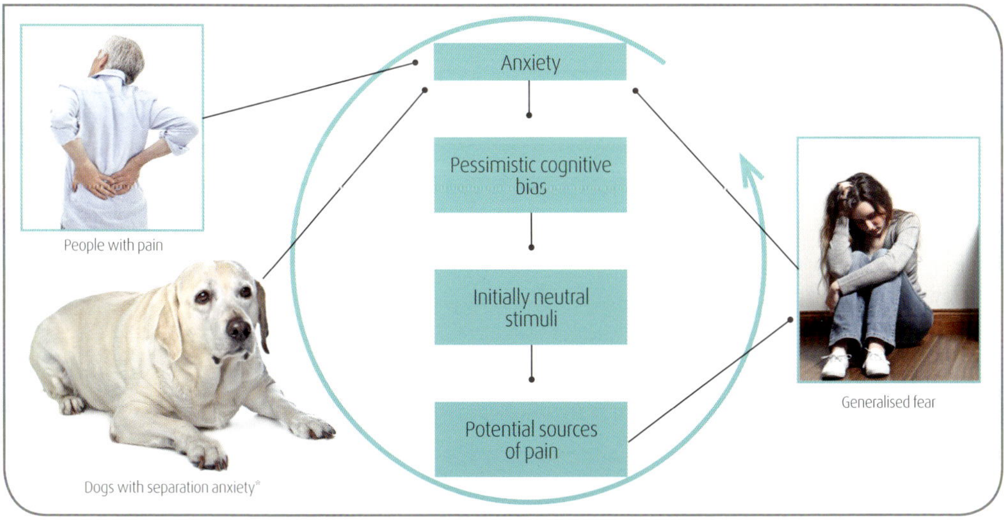

* Mendl, M., Brooks, J., Basse, C., Burman, O., Paul, E., Blackwell, E., Casey, R. Dogs showing separation-related behaviour exhibit a "pessimistic" cognitive bias. *Current Biology*, 2010; 19:839-840.

Fear problems

Epidemiology

Fear problems are very frequent, although the epidemiologic data available indicates that only 20% of dogs show problems that are serious enough for the owner to ask for a solution to a professional.

There is no epidemiological data available as regards fear problems caused or worsened by an underlying painful condition. At the Clinical Veterinary Hospital Foundation of the Faculty of Veterinary Medicine of the Autonomous University of Barcelona, treatments for animals with phobias that originated from a previous painful experience are occasionally asked for.

However, the problems derived from fear that are induced or worsened by pain are probably underestimated, especially if we take into account the fact that aggressive behaviour caused by pain has an underlying emotional fear component and could therefore be considered a fear problem.

Symptoms, diagnosis and prognosis

There is a great variety of symptoms associated with pain. Depending on the situation, the animal can freeze, try to escape, hide or even attack. In addition, depending on the intensity of the problem, other signs are observed, such as the loss of control of micturition and defecation, emptying of the anal sacs, pupil dilation, increase in the respiratory and heart rates, slight to excessive drooling, lip licking, vocalisations and frenetic attempts to escape.

The body posture (fig. 2b) of the animal when these symptoms are present helps to determine that the underlying motive is fear. The dog shows a predominantly flexed general posture, that is to say, its limbs are flexed, its back is arched and its tail is between its legs. The facial expression is also typical. Normally, the animal's ears are back, it looks away and turns its head to avoid visual confrontation. Depending on the stimulus and circumstances, it may pull its lips back to show its teeth and bite in the air or even violently attack.

The diagnosis of any fear problem is normally based on the symptoms. The elements to be taken into consideration in fear induced by pain are whether the source of pain is still present or if, on the contrary, fear is secondary to a specific painful experience.

Finally, it is important, especially for the prognosis, to know the characteristics of the parents, the experiences during the socialisation period and at the adult age. In addition, it will be necessary to describe the details of the stimuli and the circumstances that cause the problem.

The indicators of poor prognosis are:

- Chronicity.
- A deficient socialisation.
- Sharing lineage with fearful animals.
- The presence of phobic fear or generalised anxiety.
- If there is a difficulty to identify the triggering stimuli or circumstances.
- If there is a difficulty to reproduce the triggering stimuli or circumstances (e.g.: animals with fear can associate the noise of storms with atmospherical changes such as the variation of atmospheric pressure or the ozone concentration. If this is the case, the reproduction of the stimuli is very complicated and makes the treatment significantly more difficult).

Treatment

The treatment will be different depending on whether the animal is afraid of one stimulus or of specific contextual elements because of a previous painful experience, or if it has a chronic pain problem that is associated with a generalised state of anxiety.

In the first case, the animal will only show fear in the presence of stimuli that it has previously related to a painful experience. For example, when animals go to the veterinary practice, they have learnt that on one or more occasions, these stimuli have been associated with a painful experience. The animals will probably show fear in the veterinary practice, but they will not have any problems when leaving it. In these cases, the problem can be treated with the tools described next.

Behaviour modification techniques

In this case, a desensitisation and counter-conditioning programme will be considered. It consists of presenting a stimulus that initially causes a negative emotional status (fear) at the same time as offering a stimulus that produces the opposite effect to the animal (for example, a stimulus that is pleasurable to the animal). This way, after several associations, the animal will change its perception of the stimulus, which was previously negative, since the stimulus has now become a sign that a positive event is about to happen. In order to facilitate the process, counter-conditioning is associated with desensitisation, which involves presenting the stimulus gradually, that is to say, the intensity of the stimulus is initially very low and is progressively increased with time.

The example described on the next page can be extrapolated to many other daily situations in the clinic, for example, handling the animal for imaging tests, otoscopic examinations, administering subcutaneous injections, etc. However, the animal needs to be taken to the clinic only to carry out these exercises and in addition, they need to be performed when the animal is healthy. In other words, these techniques cannot be used in animals that require an emergency treatment. It can be extrapolated, however, to situations out of the clinical environment, such as for example, fear of people caused by a previous painful experience, fear of cars because of an accident, or any acute situation that has caused pain to the animal and generated a fear reaction to the stimuli that were present when pain occurred.

Finally, in the cases where a painful clinical procedure needs to be carried out, the best alternative will be the use of analgesics (see chapter 2), that can be combined with anxiolytics so that the visit to the vet is more relaxed (see below). In some cases the complete sedation of the animal will be required.

PRACTICAL EXAMPLE: NAIL TRIMMING FOR DOGS

Dogs, especially small ones, often require nail trimming. In many cases they show signs of fear during this procedure. In order to prevent this problem, the treatment consists in the following steps.

STEP 1

In these cases, counter-conditioning is done with two people and starts by placing the dog on the lap of one of them, who could be sitting on a chair. In this situation, the dog is given several rewards. While the animal is trying to take and eat them, the assistant touches the animal's paws. If the animal shows no fear reaction, we take the hand that has touched the dog away and then we take away the rewards. This should be done several times.

STEP 2

Next, we should follow the same methodology as in the previous step, that is to say, while the dog is being given some food and is paying attention to it, we take its paw with one hand. This step should be repeated several times.

STEP 3

We should then repeat the same action as before, but while holding the dog's paw with one hand, we repeatedly touch its nails with a nail clippers. This should be done several times.

STEP 4

We do the same as before, but this time making circles around the animal's nail with the nail clippers, without cutting it. This should be done several times.

STEP 5

We do the same as before, but this time we get to cut the nail. Every time a nail is cut, more rewards than before are given.

If the animal shows signs of fear at any time, we will go a few steps back in the process and will repeat the action more times.

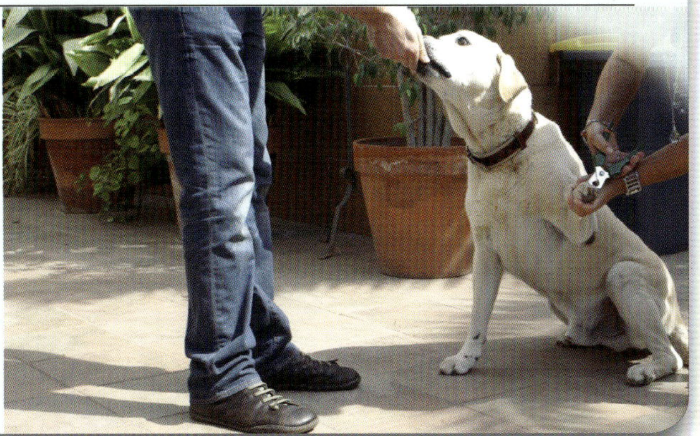

3

Use of psychoactive drugs

The use of anxiolytics in the clinic should be considered in thoses cases in which the animal already shows fear or phobia, or in those in which a very painful procedure that cannot be controlled only with analgesia needs to be carried out. The most frequently used drugs for these cases are benzodiazepines (table 2) for two reasons: firstly, because they have a short and fast-acting anxiolytic effect (depending on the type of benzodiazepine, its effect will be more or less fast and/ or long-lasting), and secondly, because benzodiazepines induce amnesia, which helps to prevent the animal from generalising the response to the painful condition to other stimuli that may be present (e.g.: the table, the vet's white coat, the smells of the room...). Benzodiazepines are GABA-boosting drugs which, as seen previously, have an inhibitory effect on fear.

Table 2. Most commonly used benzodiazepines in fear problems.

NAME	DOSE IN DOGS	DOSE IN CATS
Diazepam	0.5-2.2 mg/kg PO, according to the need	0.22-0.4 mg/kg PO, every 12-24 hours
Clorazepate	0.5-2.2 mg/kg PO, every 12-24 hours	0.125-0.25 mg/kg PO, every 12 hours
Alprazolam	0.01-0.1 mg/kg PO, every 8-12 hours	0.12-0.25 mg/kg PO, every 12 hours

In addition, they are used to make the transport of the cat to the clinic easier (also of dogs, but less frequently). Handling and transport to the clinic are thus both made easier.

The problem of benzodiazepines is that they can have a paradoxical effect. If this occurs, instead of calming down, the animal will show signs of excitement that will make the problem more difficult.

The use of some benzodiazepines (especially diazepam) is contra-indicated in cats since they can very occasionally cause acute liver failure (due to a necrosis), which is often irreversible. Acute liver failure is thought to be due to erratic metabolites produced after the first step of hepatic metabolisation after oral administration. This problem has not been described in parenteral use. In benzodiazepines that are directly conjugated, such as lorazepam and oxazepam, this problem has not been described either.

They alter the animal's cognitive abilities, which is why applying behaviour modification techniques is not recommended if the animal is under their effects, as they could drastically reduce the effectiveness of the learning sessions.

Pheromones (semiochemicals)

They are used preventively in dogs and cats to induce an anxiolytic effect, both during transport from the patient's home to the clinic and for the handling of the animal once there. Pheromones are specific to each species, and for this purpose, ther are two types available for their clinical use:

1. Dog-appeasing pheromone (semiochemical): a diffuser can be used in the waiting and examination rooms. In addition, its collar version for the animal can be used for car journeys. Several studies support their use as an anxiolytic.
2. Synthetic feline facial pheromone (semiochemical): it can be applied by means of a diffuser in the cat waiting room and examination room. Its spray presentation can be used for transport to the veterinary practice.

Nutraceuticals

The alpha-casozepine is a GABA-boosting nutraceutical, like benzodiazepines. However, although they are very safe, since no adverse effects have been described, their effects are less powerful than those of benzodiazepines.

Therapeutical approach to fear associated with chronic pain

If the animal shows a fear or anxiety problem associated with a chronic painful condition that still persists, the following elements of the treatment will vary:

- **Analgesia:** the painful condition must be controlled (see chapter 2). Both a drug treatment and measures aimed at adapting the environment to the individual needs of the animal should be applied.
- **Psychoactive drugs:** if there is a problem of generalised anxiety or fear to many stimuli, we should administer anxiolytic drugs that, in addition to ha-

ving longer-lasting effects, do not affect the animal's cognitive abilities. This way, it will be possible to use them together with behaviour modification techniques (table 3). The most commonly used drug families are:

- Tricyclic antidepressants (TCAs): they are serotonin and norepinephrine reuptake inhibitors. They are not very specific serotonergic drugs, as they also affect norepinephrine reuptake. They are antagonists of the α_1-adrenergic, antihistamine and anticholinergic receptors. The advantage of these drugs is that they are analgesic and are especially useful against neuropathic pain. Their action starts after 2-6 weeks of administration. The most used drugs in this group are clomipramine and amitryptiline.
- Selective serotonin reuptake inhibitors (SSRIs): they are very selective drugs. They are used because of their anxiolytic effect, but also for their analgesic effect. The most representative active substances in this group are fluoxetine, fluvoxamine and sertraline.
- Monoamine oxidase-A inhibitors/dopaminergic drugs: the only psychoactive drug used in this group is selegiline. This drug is used in humans against Parkinson's disease and increases dopamine levels in the CNS. It is used to treat fear problems expressed with inhibitory behaviours, but not in cases where the animal is aggressive since they can also desinhibit aggressive behaviours. In dogs, it is metabolised as L-amphetamine and L-methamphetamine, which can cause similar effects to amphetamines. Part of the desinhibitory effect that it has on fear and other behaviours, such as aggressiveness, could be due to these metabolites. They are also responsible for its side effects.
- β-blockers: in people they are mostly used to control somatic reactions to fear (sweaty and shaking hands, etc.). There are no studies available in veterinary medicine but they may be used in a few years' time. The most frequently used β-blockers are propanolol and pindolol.
- Atypical antidepressants: the most frequently used one is trazodone. It is an agonist/antagonist serotonergic drug. It also has postsynaptic antagonist effects on α_1-adrenergic receptors. It does not have any anticholinergic effects and has a moderate antihistamine activity. They are

used in veterinary medicine as adjuvants of TCAs and SSRIs. They are administered mainly in cases of generalised anxiety and fears or phobias in which the adjuvant conventional treatment with benzodiazepines has not been effective. Their effect will be limited in cases of severe phobias. When administered for several weeks, their effect is similar to that of benzodiazepines. In humans they are used mainly to eliminate the effect of SSRIs on sleep.

- α_2-agonists: clonidine is mainly used. It blocks the release of norepinephrine by activating the α_2 receptors in the presynaptic neuron, especially in the locus coeruleus. It is used for the treatment of fears and phobias (including aggressive behaviour caused by fear). It would substitute benzodiazepines in the treatment of animals with fear problems.

- **Behaviour modification techniques:** the simuli that trigger the problem or those to which the animal's fear response has generalised will need to be detailed as much as possible in order to apply a desensitisation and counter-conditioning programme.

Table 3. Most used anxiolytic drugs in dogs and cats.

GROUP OF DRUGS	DRUG	DOSE IN DOGS	DOSE IN CATS
Tricyclic antidepressants (TACs)	Clomipramine	1-3 mg/kg every 12 hours	References from 0.5 mg/kg every 24 hours, up to 1-5 mg/kg every 12-24 hours
	Amitriptyline	2.2-4.4 mg/kg every 12-24 hours	5-10 mg/cat every 24 hours, at night
	Imipramine	2-4 mg/kg every 12-24 hours	0.5-1 mg/kg every 12-24 hours
Selective serotonin reuptake inhibitors (SSRIs)	Fluoxetine	0.5-1 mg/kg every 24 hours	0.5-1 mg/kg every 24 hours, in some studies 0.5-3 mg/kg every 24-72 hours
	Paroxetine	0.5-1 mg/kg every 24 hours	1.25-2.5 mg/cat every 24 hours
	Sertraline	2.5-3.5 mg/kg every 24 hours	Not described
	Fluvoxamine	1 mg/kg every 12-24 hours	1 mg/kg every 24 hours
Atypical antidepressants	Trazodone	2.5-10 mg/kg every 24 hours	-
MAO inhibitors	Selegiline	0.5 mg/kg every 24 hours	0.5-1 mg/kg every 24 hours
α_2-agonists	Clonidine	According to the need 0.01 mg/kg once or twice a day with a maximum dose of 0.05 mg/kg twice a day, always with a minimum of 6 hours between each dose	-

SUMMARY

1. Pain acts as an unconditional stimulus in the appearance of fear.
2. The animal's response can generalise to initially neutral stimuli due to a classical conditioning process, thus worsening the problem.
3. Pain generates an anxiety response that could facilitate a pessimistic cognitive bias. At the same time, this would facilitate the animal's perception of initially neutral stimuli as possible sources of pain, and a generalisation of the fear or anxiety response would thus take place.
4. The use of learning techniques based on positive punishment induce fear in animals and should therefore be avoided.
5. The treatment will be based on both the application of behaviour modification programmes and the use of psychoactive drugs, pheromones and/or nutraceuticals.
6. The prevention of fear problems will be based on the correct breeding of the animals, through a good selection of the parents and the correct socialisation of puppies.
7. The use of analgesics and psychoactive drugs that minimise bad experiences in the clinical environment will also facilitate the prevention of the problem.

CLINICAL CASE 1

PATIENT PROFILE

9-year-old non-neutered male Labrador, weighing 42 kg.

REASON FOR CONSULTATION

The dog is examined for a problem of aggressive behaviour towards to other dog of the family and for tail chasing.

CLINICAL HISTORY

The dog was adopted from a private individual at 7 weeks of age and in a good state of health. The family is formed by a middle aged couple and a year-and-a-half-old male, non-neutered Boxer, weighing 38 kg. They live in a house with a garden and the dogs can also enter the house whenever they want if the owners are there.

The dogs go out for a walk 3 times a day for 30 minutes. They eat high-end light dry food in two rations per day (in the morning and at night). The dog's behaviour is normal with the members of the family, unknown people and unknown dogs.

The problem occurs with the other dog he lives with. They fight when the owners get home, when they eat and when they go out for a walk. The Boxer always starts the fight. The two dogs assume a defensive posture. Currently the situation is very serious, as seeing each other is enough to trigger the attack. The problem started half a year ago, when the Boxer was one year old.

The tail chasing behaviour started a few months after the Boxer arrived. It occurs in the same situations in which they fight (when they eat, when the owners arrive and sometimes when they go for a walk). The dog does it more and more often and for longer periods. Before, the owners could stop this behaviour by distracting him with food. However, now they cannot stop the behaviour, even with food.

No other significant problems have been observed as regards other aspects of the animal's behaviour.

PHYSICAL EXAMINATION AND LABORATORY TESTS

A medical check-up was carried out in order to rule out the organic diseases that most frequently can cause this type of behaviour. This check-up includes a physical examination, a neurological test and blood analysis (complete blood count and routine blood chemistry including T_4 and TSH).

During the physical examination, a wound was observed on the tip of the tail as well as pain in the sacral area. After the initial medical check-up, it was decided to carry out further tests and an X-ray and myelography were performed. A lumbosacral degenerative stenosis was diagnosed.

DIAGNOSIS

The dog showed a problem of hierarchical aggression that had worsened because of the pain derived from the lumbosacral pathology. In addition, it had a tail chasing problem that was the result of the stress caused by both the hierarchy conflict with the other dog and pain.

TREATMENT, DISCUSSION AND FOLLOW-UP

In order to try to solve the hierarchy conflict, it was recommended to neuter the Labrador, that is to say, the animal identified as submissive. Castrating the submissive dog helps to increase the distance between both individuals and therefore to settle the hierarchy. Owing to the seriousness of the problem, it was decided to administer fluoxetine to the Boxer (1 mg/kg every 24 hours, in the morning and together with food) and keep them separated. A progressive introduction was done, first by initiating the contact out of their territory 3-4 weeks after castration and after starting the drug therapy. Once their behaviour outside home was acceptable, a controlled contact was initiated inside the house. At this point it was important for the owners to give all the privileges (food, strokes, putting the leash on, etc.) first to the dominating dog and then to the subordinate one.

In order to solve the compulsive problem of tail chasing, it was necessary to eliminate the sources of stress. On the one hand, the hierarchy conflict, and on the other hand, the pain derived from the lumbosacral pathology.

Taking into accout that impredictability considerably increases stress, a walking, food and play routine is set up. In addition, we warn the owners about the importance of not reinforcing this behaviour. Punishing the dog when he is chasing his tail or distracting him with food or strokes keeps making the problem worse. The owners had to ignore the dog completely when he chased his tail. It was decided to administer clomipramine to the Labrador (initially 1 mg/kg every 12 hours, increasing to up to 3 mg/kg every 12 hours if necessary). Studies carried out in the canine species have demonstrated that this drug can be useful in the treatment of compulsive behaviour.

To reduce the pain derived from the lumbosacral pathology, carprofen was administered at a dose of 2.2 mg/kg every 12 hours, for 20 days, and then according to the evolution of the degenerative problem.

3

CLINICAL CASE 2

PATIENT PROFILE

6-year-old female Chow Chow dog, spayed, weighing 22 kg.

REASON FOR CONSULTATION

The dog is assessed for a problem of aggressive behaviour towards her owners.

CLINICAL HISTORY

She was bought from a breeder when she was 3 months old. The family is formed by 4 people, a couple and their two teenage children. They live in a flat with a terrace.

The dog goes out for a walk twice a day for 30 minutes. She used to go out 4 times a day but the owners decided to reduce the number of walks because on many occasions she refused to move when she was shown the leash.

She had never shown any aggressive behaviour before. They could touch her food when she was eating, move her away from the place where she rests, brush her, administer dosing pipettes, etc. The problem started approximately a month ago. Two events occurred over this period of time. The first one occurred when they tried to move her to go out for a walk. The dog bit the owner without any previous warning signs. The second event took place when the owner approached the animal to stroke her. At this moment, the animal started to growl and immediately bit him.

Another change that had been observed is that the dog had started to urinate in the entrance hall. This problem did not happen daily but they believed it was more and more frequent.

No other significant problems were observed as regards other aspects of the animal's behaviour.

PHYSICAL EXAMINATION AND LABORATORY TESTS

A medical check-up was carried out in order to rule out the organic diseases that most frequently cause this type of behaviour. A physical examination and blood analysis were performed (complete blood count and routine blood chemistry including T_4 and TSH).

During the physical examination, the dog reacted aggressively when the area of the hip was manipulated. A moderate dysplasia was diagnosed on the X-rays that were subsequently taken. The blood analysis was normal.

DIAGNOSIS

The dog showed a problem of aggressive behaviour caused by the pain derived from the orthopaedic problem.

TREATMENT, DISCUSSION AND FOLLOW-UP

It was recommended not to manipulate the dog or approach her when she was resting. The owners had to wait until the dog would initiate the interactions. Once the dog has gone through a painful experience (when they try to move her to go out for a walk), she can react aggressively to any similar interaction. It is a case of avoidance behaviour. The dog reacts to situations where she might get hurt by trying to avoid the "potential" painful manipulation.

In addition, it was recommended to reduce the duration of the walks (at least temporarily depending on the evolution of the orthopaedic problem) and add a third walk to prevent urination in the entrance hall. When they had to go for walk, they had to call the dog (showing her a reward if necessary) and once she would come, give her the reward. To eliminate the traces of urine and thus prevent the dog from developing an incorrect habit, it was recommended to use an enzymatic detergent for this purpose (Urine Off). At the same time, a treatment to reduce pain was initiated while the possibility of a surgery was evaluated. She was administered meloxicam, initially at a dose of 0.1 mg/kg PO, every 24 hours.

The dog did not react aggressively again.

CLINICAL CASE 3

PATIENT PROFILE

13-year-old female Siberian Husky. She was spayed at the age of 2 to avoid unwanted pregnancies. She weighs 22 kg.

REASON FOR CONSULTATION

Referred by another veterinary surgeon, with cognitive dysfunction syndrome diagnosed 2 months ago that does not improve with the measures that have been taken.

CLINICAL HISTORY

The dog was adopted from a shelter when she was one year old. She did not have any medical problems when she was adopted. According to the owners, she was the most active in the cage and they adopted her because she was the only Siberan Husky and they were looking for that breed.

She lives in 200 m^2 house with a 1,000 m^2 garden, with two middle-aged adults and no children. She can access the whole house and garden at any time. She also lives with another Siberian Husky, an 8-year-old non-neutered male, adopted at one year old when the patient was 2 (which was the reason why she was spayed).

She goes for a walk twice a day for an average 20 minutes. In fact, the walks have been reduced due to the fact that she now gets tired easily. She is usually walked with a retractable leash and a conventional collar.

She eats two rations of dry food a day and she is also randomly given homemade food as rewards.

Her elimination behaviour has changed for a few months. She used to urinate and defecate in the same specific area in the garden and now, although she still eliminates in the garden, she also does it in front of the living-room door that leads to the terrace. In addition, in the last few weeks she has not shown a normal elimination pattern and urinates and defecates in the whole garden with no specific pattern. She does not eliminate in her resting area. When she goes out for a walk, she eliminates on the pavement or on the soil, while she only did it on the soil before.

She knows basic obedience orders and nothing has changed regarding this aspect since the problem started. No obvious fears or phobias have been observed.

A few months before the consultation, she started not to sleep for the whole night. She wanders about the house and even goes out in the garden several times during the night. In the last few weeks before the visit to the vet she has been seen chasing her tail several times a day (1-3 minutes at a time). She does not bite her tail and does not show any wound on it.

The owners claim she does not seem disoriented. However, they have observed that now, when they get back gome, they can see that she has jumped up on the sofa or even on low furniture (while she had never done that before). They make a recording on our request before the consultation when the animal is alone. The dog is seen frequently wandering about the living-room, jumping up on several occasions on the sofa, where she sleeps quietly for short periods of time. She does not jump up on the furniture in the video.

SOCIAL BEHAVIOUR

Regarding the dog's behaviour with other people and animals:

- **Towards members of the family:** she has never been aggressive towards the members of the family. They have noticed that she has been paying less attention to them for a couple of years, as if she had become more independent. She wants to play neither with the owners nor with the other dog.
- **Unknown people:** the only relevant information is that the family has friends that the dog has known all her life (in fact they are the ones in charge of taking care of her when the owners are on holiday) and, however, in the last few months she has taken more time to go and greet them when she sees them, to "recognise them" (according to the owners' perception).
- **Unknown dogs:** she has always been aggressive with unknown dogs. The problem has got worse as far as intensity is concerned in the last few months. Now she does not let any dog get close to her and becomes aggressive even at a far distance. The posture is ambivalent.

CURRENT TREATMENT

On veterinary prescription, the animal has been taking selegiline (0.5 mg/kg every 24 hours, for two months) and a nutraceutical dietary supplement to slow down the clinical symptoms of brain aging, in the recommended doses.

PHYSICAL EXAMINATION AND LABORATORY TESTS

A medical check-up was carried out to rule out the organic pathologies that most frequently can cause this type of behaviour. Given the age and clinical history of the dog, this check-up included a general physical examination, a neurological examination, a complete orthopaedic examination and blood analysis (complete blood count, complete blood chemistry including total and free T_4 and TSH).

All the analytical parameters were normal, except total T_4 with a value of 1.0 µg/dl (reference values: 1.3-2.9 µg/dl). The neurological examination was normal.

Intense pain was located when extending the hip. The subsequent X-ray examination showed serious degenerative changes in both hip joints.

DIAGNOSIS AND TREATMENT

To summarise, the signs shown by the animal were:

- Alteration of the sleep-wake cycle.
- Reduced interaction with the owners.
- Reduced interaction with unknown people.
- Increase in the intensity of the aggressive behaviour towards other dogs.
- Changes in the elimination patterns.
- The dog wanders about in the house when she is alone and new behaviours, such as jumping up on the sofa (and probably on furniture), have appeared.
- Low intensity tail chasing.
- Bilateral hip joint pain.

The differential diagnosis that was established was:

- Behavioural changes related to a chronic pain problem.
- Cognitive dysfunction syndrome.
- Other medical diseases.

It was decided to perform a therapeutic test, for which the drug treatment that she was taking was progressively eliminated.

Carprofen was initially administered at a dose of 2.2 mg/kg every 12 hours for 20 days, combined with tramadol at a dose of 5 mg/kg every 8 hours, for 10 days.

No behaviour modification technique was introduced with the purpose of determining the role of pain in the overall symptoms.

FOLLOW-UP

The animal got back to her normal sleep-wake cycle 24-36 hours after the change of treatment. Her daytime activity increased as well as the interaction with both the owners and unknown people. Aggressive behaviour towards unknown dogs was maintained. The elimination pattern was still altered. Although she has stopped eliminating in front of the terrace door, the previous elimination pattern was not recovered and she kept using different areas of the garden every time (not where she used to eliminate). In the street, she continued eliminating on both the pavement and the soil. No more daytime wandering episodes were observed.

In addition to the drug treatment, several comfortable resting areas were added in the house, an anti-slip access ramp was installed on the terrace (in front of the door on the terrace that leads to the garden area of the house) and the number of street walks was increased but their duration was reduced.

Once the first step was completed, mavacoxib (2 mg/kg) was introduced in the treatment to control chronic pain, and was occasionally combined with the doses of tramadol recommended previously.

DISCUSSION

Most of the symptoms can be explained by a cognitive dysfunction problem. However, chronic hip pain could also explain the problem or worsen the symptoms of cognitive dysfunction.

The typical signs of cognitive dysfunction can be confused, as they can be very similar to those shown by some animals when they suffer from chronic pain.

- The alteration of sleep, one of the most obvious signs that is usually described by the owners of dogs with cognitive dysfunction syndrome, can be caused by chronic pain.
- The reduced interaction, both with the owners and unknown people, can also be a symptom of the dog's discomfort. The presence of pain can cause the animal to avoid stimuli that could produce more pain, such as the owners, who could unconsciously manipulate their pet in such a way that the problem would get worse, as they are not aware that she is in pain.
- Changes in the elimination pattern. Pain in the posterior third of the body could make access to certain areas of the house more difficult, a change in the elimination pattern thus being a secondary sign of this problem.
- Pain decreases the aggression threshold, it could therefore worsen the pre-exisiting problem of aggressive behaviour towards unknown dogs.
- The increase in the activity (as well as the decrease) can be explained by chronic pain. Wandering when the owners are absent could therefore also be explained by pain. However, in this case, it rather seemed to be a search for a more comfortable resting area.
- Finally, tail chasing could also be explained as a displacement behaviour caused by the stress induced both by pain and the lack of sleep.

This case highlights the need for a methodical and thorough medical check-up of all the animals that come to the practice for a behaviour problem. In these cases, the treatment of chronic pain is the first step before being able to diagnose other behaviour diseases, especially when those cannot be confirmed through complementary tests (as in cognitive dysfunction).

Bibliography

About aggressive behaviour and pain:

Association of Pet Behaviour Counsellors (APBC). Annual review of cases, 2005. United Kingdom. Available in: http://www.apbc.org.uk/

Azrin, N.H., Hutchinson, R.R., Sallery, R.D. Pain-aggression toward inanimate objects. *Journal of the experimental analysis of behavior*, 1964; vol 7:223-228.

Bardin, L. The complex role of serotonin and 5-HT receptors in chronic pain. *Behavioural Pharmacology*, 2011; vol 22:390-404.

Beaver, B.V. *Canine behavior insights and answers* (2nd ed). Saunders Elsevier, St. Louis, 2009; pp. 133-192.

Berkowitz, L., Embree, M.C. The effect of escape possibility on aversively stimulated aggression. *J Res Pers*, 1987; 21:405-416.

Berkowitz, L., Cochran, S.T., Embree, M.C. Physical pain and the goal of aversively stimulated aggression. *J Pers Soc Psychol*, 1981; 40:687-700.

Blanchard, D.C., Blanchard, R.J. Stress and aggressive behaviors. In: Nelson, R.J. (ed). *Biology of Aggression*. Oxford University Press, Inc., 2006; pp. 275-291.

Borchelt, P.L. Aggressive behavior of dogs kept as companion animals: classification and influence of sex, reproductive status and breed. *Appl Anim Ethol*, 1983; 10:45-61.

Camps, T., Amat, M., Mariotti, V.M., Le Brech, S., Manteca, X. Pain-related aggression in dogs: 12 clinical cases. *Journal of Veterinary Behavior*, 2011; in press.

Chapman, C.R., Tackett, R.P., Song, C.W. Pain and stress in a systems perspective: reciprocal neural, endocrine and immune interactions. *The Journal of Pain*, 2008; vol 9, no 2 (February):122-145.

Coccaro, E.F., Astill, J.L. Herbert, J.L., Schut, A.G. Fluoxetine treatment of impulsive aggression in DSM-III-R personality disorder patients. *J Clin Psychopharmacol*, 1990; 10:373-375.

3

Fatjó, J., Ruíz de la Torre, J.L., Manteca, X. The epidemiology of behavioural problems in dogs and cats: a survey of veterinary practitioners. *Anim Welf*, 2006; 15:179-185.

Grant, D. Pain management in small animals. *A manual for veterinary nurses and technicians*. Elsevier, UK, 2006.

Kruk, M.R., Halasz, J., Meelis, W., Haller, J. Fast positive feedback between adrenocortical stress response and a brain mechanism involved in aggressive behavior. *Behavioral Neuroscience*, 2004; 118:1062-1070.

Linthorst, A.C.E. Stress, corticotropin-releasing factor and serotonergic neurotransmission. In: T. Steckler, N.H. Kalin and J.M.H.M. Reul (eds.) *Handbook of stress and the brain*, 2005; vol. 15:503-524.

Lund, J.D., Agger, J.F., Vestergaard, K.S. Reported behaviour problems in pet dogs in Denmark: age distribution and influence of breed and gender. *Prev Vet Med*, 1996; 28:33-48.

Matsuzawa-Yanagida, K., Narita, M., Nakajima, M. et al. Usefulness of antidepressants for improving the neuropathic pain-like state and pain-induced anxiety through actions at different brain sites. *Neuropsychopharmacology*, 2008; 33:1952-1965.

McEwena, B.S., Kaliab, M. The role of corticosteroids and stress in chronic pain conditions. *Metabolism Clinical and Experimental*, 2010; 59 (Suppl 1):S9-S15.

Mehlman, P.T., Higley, J.D., Faucher, I., Lilly, A.A., Taub. D.M., Vickers, J. et al. Correlation of CSF 5-HIAA concentration with sociality and the timing of emigration in free- ranging primates. *Am J Psychiatry*, 1995; 152:907-913.

Mellor, D.J., Cook, C.J., Stafford, K.J. Quantifying some responses to Pain as a Stressor. In: Moberg, G.P., Mench, J.A. (eds.). The Biology of animal stress. *Basic principles and implications for animal welfare*. CABI Publishing, EE. UU., 2000; pp. 1.

Miczek, K.A., Fish, E.W. Monoamines, GABA, glutamate, and aggression. In: Nelson, R.J. (ed.), *Biology of aggression*. Oxford University Press, Inc. 2006; pp. 114-149.

Moyer, K.E. Kinds of aggression and their physiological basis. *Communications in Behavioral Biology*, 1968; 2:65-87.

Nelson, R.J. *Biology of Aggression*. Oxford University Press, New York, 2006.

Peremans, K., Audenaert, K., Coopman, F., Blanckaert, P., Jacobs, F., Otte, A., Verschooten, F., van Bree, H., van Heeringen, K., Mertens, J., Slegers, G., Dierckx, R. Estimates of regional cerebral blood flow and 5-HT_{2A} receptor density in impulsive, aggressive dogs with 99mTc-ECD and 123I-5-I-R91150. *Eur J Nucl Med Mol Imaging*, 2003; 30:1538-1546.

Reisner, I. An overview of aggression. In: Horwitz, D., Mills, D., Heath, S. (eds.). *BSAVA Manual of Canine and Feline Behavioural Medicine*, British Small Animal Veterinary Association, Gloucester, 2002; pp. 181-194.

Seibert, L.M., Lansdberg, G.M. Diagnosis and management of patients presenting with behavior problems. *Vet Clin Small Anim*, 2008; 38: 937-950.

Young, S.N. Some effects of dietary components (amino acids, carbohydrate, folic acid) on brain serotonin synthesis, mood and behavior. *Can J Physiol Pharmacol*, 1991; 69:893-903.

3

About compulsive behaviour and pain:

Asmundson, G.J., Katz, J. Understanding the co-occurrence of anxiety disorders and chronic pain: State-of-the-art. *Depression and Anxiety*, 2009; 26:888-901.

Luescher, A.U. Repetitive and compulsive behaviour in dogs and cats. In: Horwitz, D., Mills, D.S. (eds). *BSAVA manual of canine and feline Behavioural Medicine* (2nd ed). BSAVA, Gloucester, 2010; pp. 236-244.

Mason, G.J. Stereotypies: a critical review. *Anim Behav*, 1991; 41:1015-1037.

Schneider, B.M., Dodman, N.H., Maranda, L. Use of memantine in treatment of canine compulsive disorders. *Journal of Veterinary Behavior: Clinical Applications and Research*, 2009; 4(3):118-126.

About pain and fear, phobia and anxiety:

BAMBERGER, M., HOUPT, K.A. Signalment factors, comorbidity, and trends in behavior diagnoses in dogs: 1.644 cases (1991–2001). *J Am Vet Med Assoc*, 2006; 229(10):1591.

BEAVER, B.V. *Feline behavior: A guide for veterinarians*. W B Saunders Company, Philadelphia, 2003.

BEAVER, B.V. Canine behavior of sensory and neural origin. In: *Canine behavior: insights and answers*, 2nd ed. Saunders Elsevier, St. Louis, 2009; 2:48-107.

BLACKSHAW, J.K. Abnormal behaviour in dogs. *Aust Vet J*, 1988; 65(12):393.

BOWEN, J., Heath, S. *Behaviour problems in small animals*. Ed. Elsevier Saunders, Philadephia, 2005.

CAMPS, T., AMAT, M., MARIOTTI, V.M., LE BRECH, S., MANTECA, X. Pain-related aggression in dogs: 12 clinical cases. *Journal of Veterinary Behavior*, 2012; 7(2):99-102.

CHAPMAN, B., VOITH, V.L. Geriatric behavior problems not always related to age. *DVM*, 1987; 18(3):32.

CROWELL-DAVIS, S.C., MURRAY, T. *Veterinary psychopharmacology*. Blackwell Publishing, Ames, 2006.

DEGHANI, M., SHARPE, L., NICHOLAS, M.K. Modification of attentional biases in chronic pain patients: a preliminary study. *European Journal of Pain*, 2008; 8:585-594.

DODMAN, N.H., SHUSTER, L. *Psychopharmacology of animal behavior disorders*. Blackwell Science, Malden, Massachusetts, 1998.

DOMJAN, M. *Principios de aprendizaje y conducta*. Paraninfo, España, 2009.

JONES, R.B. Fear and distress. In: *Animal welfare*. Appleby, M.C. and Barry, O.H. (eds.). CAB International, 1997; 6:75-87.

KRUSHINSKII, L.V. Animal Behavior: Its normal and abnormal development. New York: Consultants Bureau, 1960.

LINDLEY, L. The Effects of pain on behaviour and behavioural problems part 2: Fear and anxiety. *Companion Animals*, 2012; 17:55-58.

LINDSAY, S.R. Fears and phobias. In: *Handbook of applied dog behavior and training*. Vol. 2. Etiology and assessment of behavior problems. Ed. Blackwell Publishing company, Iowa, 2001; 3:69-92.

MENDL, M., BROOKS, J., BASSE, C., BURMAN, O., PAUL, E., BLACKWELL, E., CASEY, R. Dogs showing separation-related behaviour exhibit a 'pessimistic' cognitive bias. *Current Biology*, 2010; 20(19):839-840.

TUBER, D.S., HOTHERALL, D., PETERS, M.F. Treatment of fears and phobias in dogs. *Vet Clin North Am (Small Anim Pract)*, 1982; 12(4):607.

3

COMPANION ANIMAL WELFARE AND PAIN

Definition and general concepts

Although some philosophers raised the issue of the responsibilities of human beings towards animals in the 18th century or even before that, the concern for animal welfare has undoubtedly grown considerably over the last few years. This is basically due to two statements. The first is that animals are able to experience suffering and feel pain, as thoroughly discussed in the first chapter. The second statement is that it is not morally acceptable to cause suffering to an animal, at least when there is no reason to justify such an act. As a result, the concern for animal welfare does not only depend on objective parameters, but also on the historical period and social, cultural and economic aspects.

In other words, many practices or attitudes towards animals which were accepted in the past are now completely rejected or, at least, by part of the society. In fact, this ethical or moral element of animal welfare is what makes it possible, even within the same society, to find groups of people who are in favour of certain practices and others who are totally against, as occurs with bullfighting events or other examples such as aesthetic amputations in companion animals or declawing to solve scratching problems in cats.

However, the exhaustive analysis of this ethical and moral aspect is far beyond the scope of this book, which will focus mainly on the objective analysis of animal welfare.

Definition of animal welfare

There are many different definitions of the concept of animal welfare. For example, Marian Dawkins (1988) gives a rough definition of it in emotional terms and claims that the concern for animal welfare should focus on "the absence of unpleasant feelings such as suffering and pain". Other authors, however, define this concept in a more functional way. The most well-known example of this is the definition given by Broom (1986), which claims that "the welfare of an animal is its state as regards its attempts to cope with its environment". In this latter case, negative feelings, and thus the lack of welfare, would appear as a consequence of the repeated (and unsuccessful) attempts of an animal to adapt to its environment. If we consider these definitions and many others available, there seems to be three key aspects:

1. **The suffering of animals:** to guarantee good welfare, situations which can cause any type of suffering to the animal, such as fear and pain, should be avoided.
2. **Environment:** depending on the environment, the animal will adapt more or less easily to it. Three scenarios can take place (fig. 1). In the first scenario, the animal is not able to adapt to the environment and thus dies. The second scenario is that of an environment to which the animal can easily adapt, without "making any effort". Finally, the last situation is that to which the animal can adapt, but at a cost. This cost will be reflected in the consequences that the generated stress response (especially if it is chronic) may have on the animal, and in the possible negative consequences of the behavioural changes shown by the animal. In other words, to guarantee the welfare of an animal, its environment should have the elements necessary to make adaptation easy.
3. **Natural behaviours:** the third element refers to the natural behaviours of animals which are important in themselves. In short, if the animal is not able to carry out these behaviours in the domestic environment, this will again cause a stress response as well as behavioural changes that may be harmful to the animal.

Figure 1. Welfare as the degree of adaptation to the environment.

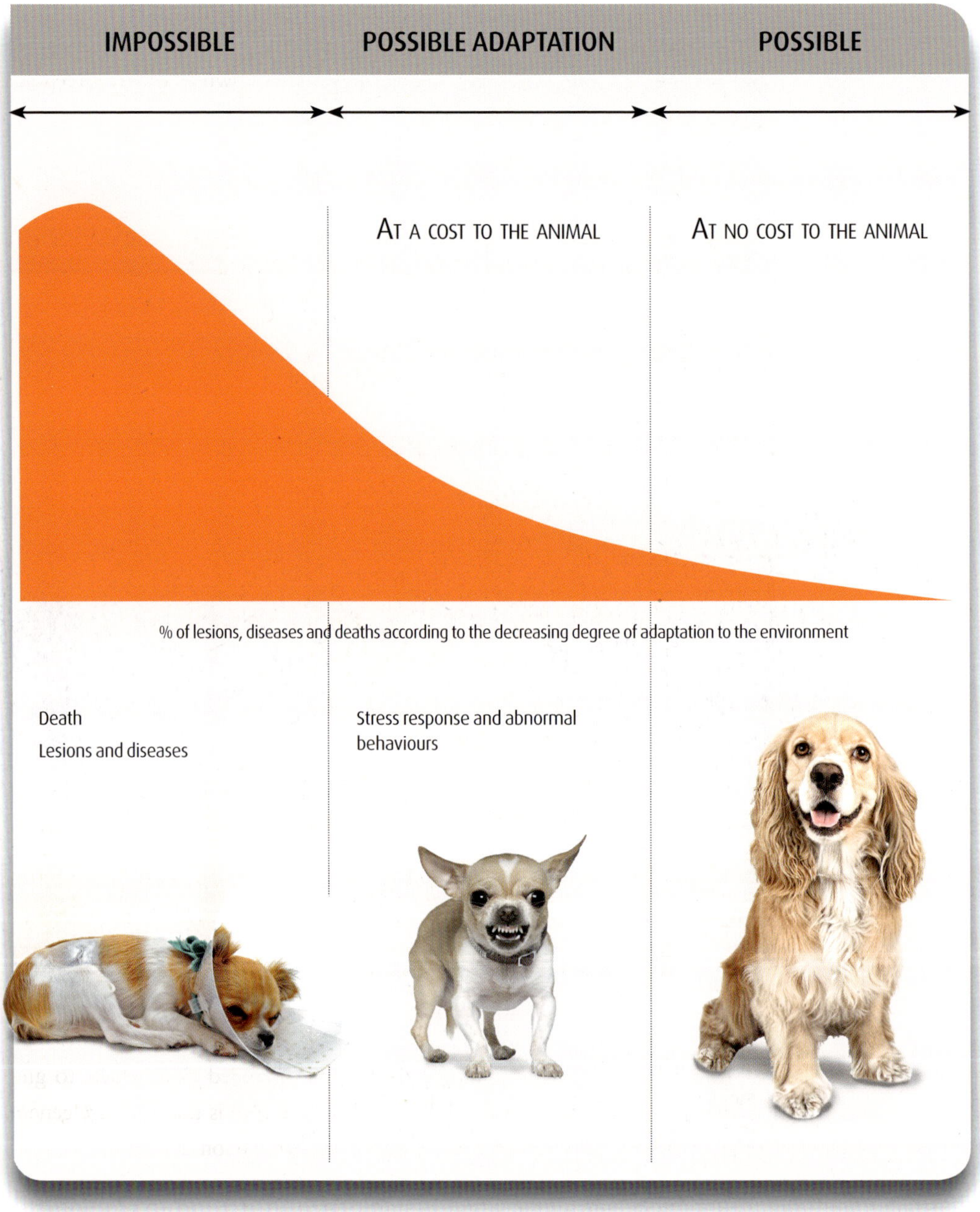

In an attempt to simplify and put all these elements together, the Farm Animal Welfare Council, a consulting organ of the British government on farm animal welfare-related issues, proposed that animal welfare is guaranteed when five requirements are met. These requirements are known as the five freedoms (see table).

THE FIVE FREEDOMS

1. Freedom from hunger and thirst.
2. Freedom from pain, injury or disease.
3. Freedom from discomfort.
4. Freedom from fear or distress.
5. Freedom to express normal behaviour.

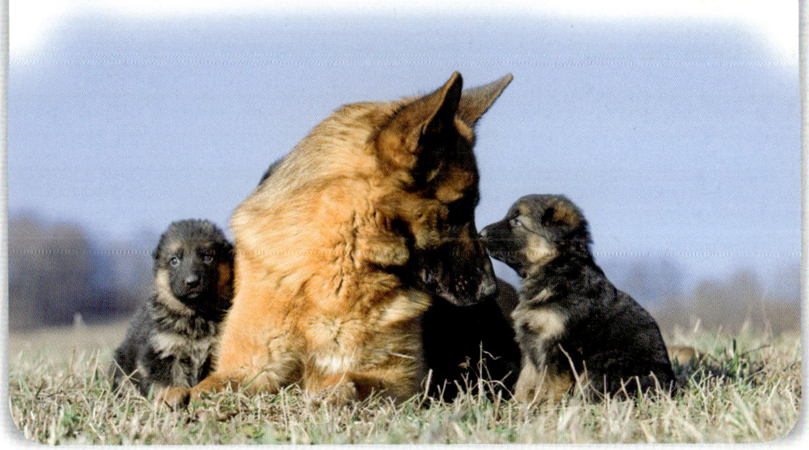

Although the five freedoms were initially formulated as a vehicle to guarantee animal welfare in production animals, the truth is that they are general enough to be applied to other animals, such as companion animals.

4

Pain and welfare

The relationship between pain and the lack of welfare goes beyond the second freedom, which claims explicitly that the presence of pain affects animal welfare. In other words, pain can affect welfare indirectly, basically through the following paths:

- **Pain and fear:** the relationship between pain and fear has been discussed in detail in chapter 3. Even though the initial cause of pain may disappear, if this pain has generated a fear response in the animal and this is maintained in a chronic manner, welfare will also be jeopardised (fourth freedom: freedom from fear or distress). Therefore, both pain and the possible associated fear response need to be treated.
- **Pain and stress:** both acute and chronic pain can induce negative affective states such as anxiety. These negative affective states, as the five freedoms describe, should be avoided to guarantee animal welfare. Once again, and in a different way, pain directly affects the level of welfare shown by an animal.
- **Pain and aggressiveness:** as seen in previous chapters, pain can bring about aggressive behaviours through different mechanisms. However, all of them have in common the fact that these aggressive behaviours favoured by pain lead to a stress response in the animal. Pain, stress and aggressiveness all feed on each other and, in any case, directly affect the state of welfare of the animal.
- **Pain and repetitive behaviours:** both carrying out abnormal behaviours, e.g. stereotypies, and the inability to show other normal behaviours, such as play or interaction with the environment or other individuals, indicate welfare problems. There is a double relationship between pain, stereotyped behaviour and welfare. On the one hand, pain can cause stress and thus trigger compulsive behaviour. Such behaviour is considered an indicator of the lack of well-being and its mere presence could therefore indicate a welfare problem. On the other hand, it must be taken into account that any repeated behaviour prevents the animal from expressing other behaviours that could be considered necessary or positive and, as a result, its welfare may indirectly be affected.

- **Pain and diseases:** there is much evidence, in many different species, of the relationship between stress and certain diseases - among which are found autoimmune diseases, certain types of cancer, heart problems or alterations of eating habits - as well as of its negative effects on ageing, memory, gastrointestinal transit, etc. If we consider pain as a potential source of chronic stress, then the relationship between pain and these diseases represents another indirect way in which welfare can be affected.

The accumulative nature of stress should also be highlighted. This means that various sources of stress increase the intensity of the response or make it last longer. This, in addition to processes such as hyperalgesia or allodynia, which were explained in previous chapters, and their direct effect on the animal's welfare, turn pain into a need for treatment, since it is another source of stress that could be added to other possible stressful situations that the animal may be underdoing.

New approaches to welfare

At its beginnings, and for many years, the study of animal welfare focused on how to avoid those negative situations or experiences for the animal. In fact, of the five freedoms, the first four focus on negative concepts (avoiding pain, hunger, stress, thermal or physical discomfort, etc.) and the fifth one on the ability to express normal behaviour. However, none of them explicitly mentions the value that the presence of positive experiences could have on animal welfare.

Over the last few years, research on welfare has mainly focused on the implication of positive behaviours rather than on the absence of negative ones, which are already well categorised. Some authors, such as Broom (1996), Webster (2005), Dawkins (2006), Boissy et al. (2007) or Morton (2007), have included concepts such as "happiness", or what the animal "wants" or "likes" in the study of welfare and have started to analyse their impact on animal welfare.

In other words, what the animal "feels" (its welfare) can vary within a range. It is not an "all or nothing" concept. In a very simplified way, it could be said that an animal with poor welfare is an animal that is suffering (from pain, thermal discomfort, fear, etc.), and an animal with good welfare is an animal that is "happy". However, there is a large gap between being happy and suffering. Animals that are neither suffering nor happy would be somewhere in between this range and would be animals whose needs (the five freedoms) are met. Some authors call these animals "content animals".

The concept of the five freedoms, which is still valid and very useful, is not contradicted by these arguments, but it becomes evident that these criteria are incomplete and that the study of animal welfare will include both concepts in a near future.

SUMMARY

- Although the concern for animal welfare is not recent, it has greatly increased in the last decades. Furthermore, significant progresses have been made in its objective study.
- The concept of the five freedoms is a useful approach, which is globally accepted as a way of guaranteeing animal welfare.
- The second freedom explicitly requires the absence of pain to guarantee animal welfare.
- In addition, pain can indirectly affect welfare. For instance, by causing a fear response, aggressive or stereotyped behaviours, medical problems, or by preventing normal and positive behaviours to the animal, such as social contact and play.
- The study of welfare has recently been extended by incorporating concepts such as "happiness", in an attemp to evaluate the presence of positive feelings in the animal.

Bibliography

Boissy, A., Arnaud, C., Chaillou, E., Desire, L., Duvaux-Ponter, C., Leterrier, C., Richard, S., Roussel, S., Saint-Dizier, H., Meunier-Salaün, M.C., Balance, D., Veissier, I. Emotions and cognitions: a new approach to animal welfare. *Animal Welfare*, 2007; 16(S):37-43.

Boissy, A., Manteuffel, G., Jensen, M.B., Moe, R.O., Spruijt, B., Keeling, L.J., Winckler, C., Forkman, B., Dimitrov, I., Langbein, J., Bakken, M., Veissier, I., Aubert, A. Assessment of positive emotions in animals to improve their welfare: Review. *Physiology and behavior*, 2007; 92:375-397.

British Veterinary Association, Animal Welfare Foundation (BVA AWF), 2006. What makes my pet happy? (leaflet). Available in: www.bva-awf.org.uk/resources/downloads.

Broom, D.M. Indicator of poor welfare. *British Veterinary Journal*, 1986; 142:524-526.

Broom, D.M. Animal welfare: the concept of the issues. In: Dollins, F.L. (ed.), *Attitudes to animals*. Cambridge University Press, Cambridge, 1999; pp. 129-142.

Dawkins, M.S. Behavioural deprivation: a central problem in animal welfare. *Applied Animal Behaviour Science*, 1988; 20:209-225.

Dawkins, M.S. Through animal eyes: what behaviour tells us. *Applied Animal Behaviour Science*, 2006; 100:4-10.

Macpherson, C.N.L., Meslin, F.X., Wandeler, A.I. (eds.). Preface in *Dogs, zoonoses and public heatlh*. CABI publishing, Wallingford, UK, 2000; pp. XI-XIII.

Mellor, D.J., Cook, C.J., Stafford, K.J. Quantifying some responses to pain as a stressor. In: Moberg, G.P., Mench, S.A. (eds.). *The biology of animal stress. Basic principles and implications for animal welfare*. CABI Publishing, USA, 2000; pp. 171-198.

4

ROCHLITZ, I. *The welfare of cats*. Ed. Springer, Netherlands, 2007.

STAFFORD, K. *The welfare of dogs*. Ed. Springer, Netherlands, 2007.

YEATES, J.W., MAIN, D.C.J. Assessment of positive welfare: A review. *The Veterinary Journal*, 2008; 175:293-300.

YEATES, J.W. Maximising canine welfare in veterinary practice and research: A review. *The Veterinary Journal*, 2011; In press doi: 10.016/j.tvjl.2011.10.024.

WEBSTER, J. *Animal welfare: limping towards Eden*. Blakwell, Oxford, 2005.

Photo credits

Shutterstock.com:

Title page: WilleeCole (dog), sheelamohanachandran2010 (neuron synapse).

Chapter 1: Page 33 (column by column); Eric Isselée, Smileus, Eric Isselée, Eric Isselée, Tony Wear, Susan Schmitz, bonchan, Pakhnyushcha, Sergii Figurnyi, Stefan Petru Andronache, Eric Isselée, Svetlana Mihailova, Tsekhmister, Eric Isselée, Sascha Burkard, Paul Hakimata Photography.

Chapter 2: Page 69; Alaettin YILDIRIM (fig. 1), Shonn (fig. 2), ktynzq (fig. 3).

Chapter 3: Page 79; Erik Lam. Page 88; Michael Pettigrew. Page 98 (line by line); Nixx Photography, Evgeny Dubinchuk, Gorilla, Sinelyov, Yuri Arcurs, Volodymyr Krasyuk, Eric Isselée (also on page VI), Kirill Vorobyev (also on page VI). Page 105; wavebreakmedia ltd, Erik Lam, Darrin Henry.

Chapter 4: Page 134; cynoclub, Eric Isselée, Susan Schmitz. Page 135; Lenkadan.

Published by Servet editorial - Grupo Asís Biomedia S.L.